Group Therapy for High-Conflict Divorce

The "No Kids in the Middle" (Kinderen uit de Knel) intervention programme addresses high-conflict divorce through a multi-family approach. This first English language edition contains descriptions of the therapeutic sessions, references to a workbook (van der Elst et al., in press) for parents and their network, along with extra information about the theoretical foundations of the programme.

The book starts with theoretical foundations and a summary of the scientific research behind the methodology before moving on to focus on the methodology of the intervention programme per session, with detailed descriptions of each therapeutic session. Through these session descriptions, the authors demonstrate how the theory of the methodology can be put into practice within a group setting. The methodology is also conveyed in such a way that the key pillars and themes are clear, with a best-practice framework clearly demonstrated. Yet at the same time, the authors leave room for customization depending on the actual clients and therapists, and for this framework to be built upon further.

With this programme now practiced and studied throughout Europe, *Group Therapy for High-Conflict Divorce* and it's methodology will act as a living framework to help continuously improve practice and research among professional therapists, while also appealing to social workers and legal professionals.

Margreet Visser is a clinical psychologist/psychotherapist and senior researcher at The Children's Trauma Center (KJTC) Kenter Jeugdhulp in the Netherlands. She is specialized in working with traumatized children and their families. Her research focusses on the impact of destructive parental conflicts on children and their families.

Justine van Lawick is a clinical psychologist, family therapist and co-founder of the Lorentzhuis. She is a senior trainer in the Netherlands and abroad.

"This book provides an incredibly comprehensive, yet rich and sophisticated guide to working with families using the No Kids in the Middle programme. van Lawick and Visser describe the innovative approach and its theoretical underpinnings with clarity, while sensitively addressing the many complexities of working with high conflict separated parents and their children. In the same way that the program aims to help parents, this book will help professionals to see new possibilities for approaching familiar difficulties and finding new solutions with the families they support."

Emma Morris, *Consultant Clinical Psychologist, Anna Freud National Center for Children and Families, London*

"This positive and creative contribution is the culmination of years of endeavour and practice by experienced therapists and clinicians in the complex arena of conflictual divorce and its consequences for children and their families. It stands as a shining example of effective practice that counteracts the ongoing unproductive conflicts between family members and their networks. In van Lawick and Visser's approach, children become allies to change, rather than victims of conflict between parents, and their voices are strengthened through group participation. The elegance of this approach is how, in time, parents listen, hear, and are moved by the words of their children and become prepared to respond in more constructive ways as they try to manage life after divorce. The No Kids in the Middle programme is an expression of hope, creativity and resilience that deserves to be promoted widely in organizations offering a post divorce service particularly where adversarial approaches have failed to reach a liveable resolution for all involved."

Jim Wilson, *UKCP Systemic Family Therapy supervisor, author and international trainer in family therapy*

"When children get caught up right in the middle of their parents' chronic and acrimonious conflicts, their mental health is often severely compromised. Creative and effective, this highly innovative approach puts children back in the centre of parental concerns. Essential reading for therapists and parents alike!"

Eia Asen, *Professor, Anna Freud Centre and University College London*

Group Therapy for High-Conflict Divorce

The "No Kids in the Middle" Intervention Programme

Margreet Visser and
Justine van Lawick

Routledge
Taylor & Francis Group
LONDON AND NEW YORK

First published in English 2021, by Routledge
2 Park Square, Milton Park, Abingdon, Oxon OX14 4RN

and by Routledge
52 Vanderbilt Avenue, New York, NY 10017

Routledge is an imprint of the Taylor & Francis Group, an informa business

Translated by Roelie Dröge-Bouwers

First Dutch edition published by SWP 2014

Second Dutch edition published by SWP 2015

Third Dutch edition published by SWP 2019

British Library Cataloguing-in-Publication Data
A catalogue record for this book is available from the British Library

Library of Congress Cataloging-in-Publication Data
A catalog record for this book has been requested

ISBN: 978-0-367-10922-6 (hbk)
ISBN: 978-0-367-10923-3 (pbk)
ISBN: 978-0-429-02391-0 (ebk)

Typeset in Times New Roman
by Apex CoVantage, LLC

Contents

Preface

The No Kids in the Middle programme was born out of discontent with the results of treatments of parents and/or children in very complicated divorce situations, also called high-conflict divorces. Results often failed to materialize or appeared to be unsatisfactory. In the Lorentzhuis centre for systemic therapy, training and consultation, several experienced system therapists and trainers get caught up in the destructive battle of divorced parents. Often, what is effective in relational therapy seems not to work here. Distrust, paranoia and a defensive attitude seriously frustrate or stand in the way of a safe therapeutic relationship, which is essential for effective psychotherapy. What complicates matters is the "juridification" of the battle: parents are all too quick to threaten to file a lawsuit, a complaint or to start summary proceedings.

At the KJTC (Children's Trauma Centre), experienced therapists struggle with the other side of the same medal: they receive many applications for treatment of children who turn out to be caught up in the high-conflict divorce of their parents. They show a wide variety of complaints and symptoms. The KJTC will continue to have difficulty treating these children properly if the context does not change. Psychotherapy may even aggravate the children's complaints: the children start to become even more aware of how deeply they are caught up in a destructive and powerless position. They learn to express themselves in therapy, whilst at home, of all places, they cannot express their pain just because all utterances could be used as ammunition in the parental conflict. The KJTC has come to conclude that the focus should be on the parents, as they are the ones to first create a safe context for their children again.

That is how the Lorentzhuis and the KJTC found each other and started to successfully cooperate in developing a programme for parents in a high-conflict divorce and their children, called No Kids in the Middle.

Beginning in early 2012, we have gained experience with a new method of working, which is described in this book as the No Kids in the Middle methodology. A central feature of this methodology is that the parents and their children are treated in groups. The experience gained so far is promising and has inspired us to extend the programme. No Kids in the Middle has become a permanent offering at both the KJTC and the Lorentzhuis. In the meantime, teams have been trained and treatment is provided in many places in the Netherlands. The programme is now even offered in various countries in Europe with locally trained teams.

Children are our guide. They teach us what it is all about: that parents stop blaming and demonizing each other, that their attention should be on the children and that they should treat each other with kindness.

On the English edition

Since the second edition appeared in 2015, the No Kids in the Middle programme has continued to evolve. That is why the book has been revised and expanded on a number of points. New insights have been incorporated throughout the book. The keystones, which are the basis of the programme, have been worked out and described more elaborately. This translated third edition also deals with the indications and contraindications of the programme. We have added a chapter about the scientific study conducted between 2012 and 2018. Finally, the programme for the children's group has been worked out in more detail.

An important development in the No Kids in the Middle programme is the *Group Therapy for High-Conflict Divorce: A Workbook for the "No Kids in the Middle" Intervention Programme.*[1] The workbook contains home assignments for all sessions, with many additional assignments, exercises and more in-depth text. Chapter 8 of this edition describes the sessions of the parent group. Each session ends with a section called "Get moving", which refers to the homework for parents and their networks. The homework is described in the workbook. The workbook and Chapter 8 of this book are therefore inseparable.

We expect all parents who are going to join the programme to use the workbook. The workbook can be a great support for parents and therefore also for the therapists. Depending on local funding of the No Kids in the Middle programme, parents will receive the workbook for free or they will have to pay for it themselves.

No Kids in the Middle® is a registered trademark

The name No Kids in the Middle is linked to our methodology and may only be used after having followed the training.[2] The training consists of three days of training, plus a minimum of six hours of supervision for the team, preferably divided into three sessions of supervision the first time the group intervention is offered. This is because we want to make sure that those offering the programme have been well-trained in the child-oriented and systemic approach and will benefit from our experiences while carrying out the complex work with these families.

Notes

1 van der Elst, E., Wierstra, J., van Lawick, J. & Visser, M., (in press), *Group Therapy for High-Conflict Divorce: A Workbook for the "No Kids in the Middle" Intervention Programme*.
2 See www.kinderenuitdeknel.nl or www.nokidsinthemiddle.com

Acknowledgements

We would like to thank all the colleagues who have contributed so far to the development, implementation and fine-tuning of the programme. In particular, Erik van der Elst, Jeroen Wierstra, Flora van Grinsven, Elisabeth van der Heide Wendy de Visser and Angela Andriesse.

We also thank the teams of the KJTC and the Lorentzhuis who had to adjust but stayed positive anyway, and helped us deal with the practical problems we ran into during the first years. We also thank all the teams, in and outside the Netherlands, for the continuous dialogue about the programme. The dialogue between providers, parents, children, scientists and policymakers helps the No Kids in the Middle programme to continuously get better.

We thank the sponsors who made it possible for us to develop the programme and conduct research into it: Meindert de Hoop Stichting, Stichting Achmea Slachtoffer en Samenleving and Stichting Kinderpostzegels. We thank the Ministry of Health, Welfare and Sports for enabling us to write this book and to sustain the programme.

Then, there is Evelyn Wilms. She volunteered to take charge of the waiting list and the administration. Her initiative led to securing grant funding to sustain the No Kids in the Middle programme. And, thanks to her, the funding is now optimally used and she has become our coordinator. Thank you so much, Evelyn! We would also like to thank the board of the No Kids in the Middle foundation, who encourage and support us and always make sure that developments and finances are properly accounted for. Of course, we thank Niels and Arthur, our beloved partners, who have actively supported us in writing this book. Especially Niels, who has made himself indispensable with his painstaking editing and his creative artwork.

But most of all, we thank all the parents who have participated and are going to participate in our programme and help us figure out what does and doesn't work. In particular, we wish to thank all the children who participated and will be participating in the programme for their efforts, their resilience and hope. They help us carry on and keep on searching for a better way.

Margreet Visser and Justine van Lawick

Chapter 1

Introduction

In the Netherlands, 86,000 children each year experience parental divorce (Voert, 2019). Forty to forty-five per cent of the children in the US go through the divorce of their parents before the age of 18 (Schoen & Canudas-Romo, 2006). Each year between 1960 and 2010, the number of divorces increased in Europe and in the US. In 2010, there was a slight decrease in most countries. In the US, divorce figures are still higher than in any European country, although divorce figures in Belgium, Switzerland, Czech Republic and Lithuania almost reach those of the US (Amato, 2014).

In most divorces (approximately 70%) parents handle the aftermath of the divorce reasonably well to well (Whiteside, 1998; Whiteside & Becker, 2000). Partners can make an arrangement to sustain the quality of life of both themselves and their children. Recent research has shown that although children may be bothered by the many changes and necessary adjustments, most of them are doing well after some time and also in the long run. They feel that they really matter to their parents and that they remain central, despite the emotional and other problems resulting from the divorce. Accordingly, these children do not function differently from those of parents who stay together (Buysse et al., 2011; Hughes, 2005).

Children appear to suffer most from battling parents, whether they live together or not. In 30 per cent of divorce cases there are financial problems and/or problems with the parenting plan. In 15 per cent of this group, the divorces proceed in a very problematic way (Spruijt & Kormos, 2014). International research shows that approximately eight to 12 per cent of the parents remain caught up in serious conflicts, even up to two to three years after the divorce (Kelly & Emery, 2003).

This is the group of parents we deal with in this programme. The divorce is a long and dragging process, full of destruction, revenge, paranoia and demonization. In some cases, parents have never lived together, but they do share custody of their child(ren) and continuously fight over care and parental access. In these destructive processes, children get caught up and damaged (Spruijt & Kormos, 2014). In the Netherlands, each year, an additional 3,000 children become victims of these divorced, battling parents. A report of the children's ombudsman (Dullaert, 2014) states that around 16,000 children suffer from their parents' high-conflict divorce. For some of them, there is no end to it and the damage continues into adulthood.

These are shocking figures, especially when you consider that there is a strong association between parental conflicts and psychosocial problems in children, such as anxiety, depression and aggressive behaviour (Amato & Cheadle, 2005; Amato & Keith, 1991). Additionally, the more serious the parental conflicts surrounding a divorce, the more serious the psychosocial consequences for the children (Amato, 2001; Amato & Keith, 1991).

High-conflict divorces are characterized by long-lasting conflict, animosity, guilt, emotional instability and the inability of partners to take responsibility for their part in the fights (Anderson et al., 2010). These characteristics lead to a cycle of negativity which can escalate (Ridley, Wilhelm & Surra, 2001). Middelberg (2001) calls this pattern the "dance of conflict", which is characterized by accusations, criticism, a lack of empathy for the other person, emotional reactivity, and a cycle of attack and counterattack.

Since parents in high-conflict divorces show little and often even a total lack of consideration for the impact of their conflicts on the children, the high-conflict divorce can be considered to be a form of emotional abuse (Dalton, Carbon & Olesen, 2003; van Lawick, 2012). After all, high-conflict divorces feature several aspects of emotional child abuse (e.g. exposure to humiliation, verbal violence, intimidation, social isolation, threats, rejection) and emotional neglect (e.g. lack of availability and supervision, failing to protect the child against emotional damage, not responding to the needs of the child).

Davies, Winter and Cicchetti (2006) point out that interparental violence affects the children in two ways, both directly and indirectly. The battle affects children's lives directly because children see and hear the conflicts, or are part of them. This immediately evokes feelings, thoughts and behaviour. Interparental conflicts also affect children indirectly. They may lead to deteriorated parenting and parent-child relationships (Buehler & Gerard, 2002). Children are also indirectly affected in the sense that the amount of time and money spent on the battle, including on the legal battle, in addition to the psychological burden of the battle on the parents leads to them being less available for their children. So even if parents manage to keep their children away from their conflicts, there is an indirect effect in terms of less parental availability for the children as a result of the continuing spiral of conflict, emotional exhaustion and fewer financial resources.

So it will not be a surprise that many children exposed to interparental violence experience stress when they are exposed to the divorce battle of their parents. The most common reactions of children exposed to interparental violence are sadness, anxiety, anger and powerlessness (Pels, Lünnemann & Steketee, 2011). If the battle continues (also after the separation of the parents), children often develop psychosocial problems and can get traumatized. They may develop symptoms such as concentration problems, hyperactivity, somatic complaints, depression, loneliness, anxiety, over-adjusting behaviour, learning problems, suicide attempts, and aggressive and oppositional behaviour (Bream & Buchanan, 2003; Dalton, Carbon & Olesen, 2003; Jaffe, Crooks & Poisson, 2003; Kelly & Emery, 2003).

The No Kids in the Middle programme has been developed for these children, their parents and their networks, and this book is intended for them.

Reader's guide

The book consists of two parts:

Part 1 covers the theory and consists of the theoretical basis (Chapter 2) and the results of the scientific study (Chapter 3). The study results have been incorporated into the methodology.

Part 2 deals with practice and describes the methodology. Chapter 4 outlines the structure of the programme and elaborates on safety issues. Chapter 5 describes the keystones. Then follows a description of intake and indication (Chapter 6), the network meeting (Chapter 7), the sessions of the parent group (Chapter 8) and those of the children's group (Chapter 9).

Part 1

Theory and research

Chapter 2

Theoretical basis[1]

2.1 Escalating conflicts

High-conflict divorces are characterized by ever-escalating conflicts. The conflict escalation ladder of Glasl (2001) shows that conflicts tend to harden. In an early stage, which he labels the rational stage, there is still room for agreement. Both parties are still able to work things out properly. When the conflict does not result in a solution, parties end up in the emotional stage, stage 2. Emotions get on top and other people are drawn into the conflict. Two networks start to fight each other. A neutral position is no longer feasible. People often find it hard to work things out without help. When the conflict continues, it will end up in a fight, stage 3. The battling parties get embittered and the battle is getting more and more fierce. The parties involved are locked in their tunnel vision and are no longer able to see things in perspective and to reflect upon themselves. The other person becomes an opponent who has to be defeated with all means available. Together into the abyss, even at the cost of life.

This theory has been developed for organizations, but can also be applied to divorce issues. Numerous mediators use the theory as a basis. At the same time, this theory suggests that conflicts neatly move from stage 1 into stage 2 and then into stage 3. Practice, however, has taught us something different. Parents can skip stages 1 and 2 and directly dive into stage 3 with their conflicts. Sometimes this happens before the divorce, sometimes at the time of the divorce and sometimes only years after the divorce. Conflicts in stage 3 can arise after an incident which triggers such intense emotions in the parties involved that things are no longer controllable from that point onwards. Fighting is the only option left. And sometimes conflicts go back from stage 3 into stage 1 if both parents have, for instance, met new partners who help them calm down. Many policymakers hope they can prevent things by recognizing when parents are in stage 1, or are moving from stage 1 into stage 2 in enough time so they can de-escalate well in advance. Unfortunately, reality is much more stubborn.

To date, the No Kids in the Middle programme has mainly focussed on stage 3, high-conflict divorces. Parent couples who are caught up in an emotional battle (stage 2) are also eligible for the programme. For these couples, too, a group approach is an appropriate and effective way to stop the battle.

2.2 Typical factors of high-conflict divorces

High-conflict divorces are characterized by six groups of interrelated and interacting factors:

1 *Demonization and rising stress*
Parties demonize each other. This process of demonization causes continuous stress and emotional reactions, externalizing and/or internalizing. Stress, escalating conflicts and destructive communication patterns dominate interactions. With parents having tunnel vision of their own convictions and their own monologue, there is no room for listening, contemplation, reflection, empathy and dialogue. These dynamics are related to the vulnerability cycle (see section 2.2.1). Parents are triggered in their vulnerability and launch into their survival strategy, which will trigger the very vulnerability of the other person.
2 *Active role of the social network*
Many have become involved in the battle. Not only the children, but also the wider social network, from grandparents, new partners, children and relatives of the new partners, friends, neighbours, lawyers, mediators, social workers, and the GP to school and work. It is not just two people fighting, it is two communities fighting each other.
3 *Arguing about the divorce story and about goals*
There is no end to the divorce story and it develops into a fight about wishes, goals and what needs to be done.
4 *Children falling off the radar*
Children, their development and well-being fall off the radar, both in their own family circle and the wider circle of professionals.
5 *Sense of powerlessness*
The parents and children involved feel powerless, but so do the people in the private and professional network around them.

6 *Stagnated transition*
The transition from being together to being separated is not made. A high-conflict divorce is a failed divorce. Parents continue to be closely involved with each other.

2.2.1 Demonization and rising stress

Demonization is a common thing among divorced parents who continue to fight. The other person is the demon who makes things difficult, destroys and ruins everything. The process of demonization is linked with the inability to accept the tragedy of life (Alon & Omer, 2005). We live in a society where the illusion that everything can be achieved and created dominates. If something does not feel right or does not meet the expectations, then something has to be changed or repaired. The other, the child, the circumstances, the therapist, the lawyers, the law and so on. Since there is always a factor outside the person itself that needs to be changed, energy and emotions will be targeted at the other factor. And if the other factor is not about to change, frustration and emotions run high. The parents involved fail to accept that tragedy and frustration are a fact of life. They keep trying to change the other person, the other factor, with ever-increasing rage.

Divorce, if there are also children involved, is a life-changing event. Parents have to give up on the romantic idea that they will grow old and raise the children together or will even have more children and, later, grandchildren together. They find themselves in a mourning process, in which black-and-white thinking about the other seems to help them mourn and deal with the divorce. Boss (2006) speaks of ambivalent mourning: the other is lost, is no longer available, but is still there. Most parents are able to keep the necessary distance after some time. They pick up their lives again, leave the black-and-white world and can face each other again with different colours. They can even start to see the other's good sides again. Parents who are caught up in a continuous battle seem to be stuck in dealing with the divorce. This causes stress and is why parents continue to only see each other's negative sides and keep having polarized ideas about each other.

Since this demonization in high-conflict divorces is mutual, communication will always escalate into conflicts. The stress system is continuously activated and stress keeps building – stress as a result of continuous fighting, stress about seeing or not seeing the children, stress about legal cases, about money issues, about the parenting schedule, about the house, loss of relatives, in-laws, friends, neighbours and stress related to mourning about the divorce.

When parents separate and there are differences of opinion about the parental schedule and other plans, it is all the more important that they are able to properly listen to each other, to be flexible and to make concessions. It is important that they can empathize with each other and with their children. This enables them to balance different interests and to see each other's positive and negative sides. They have to be able to deal with frustrations and trust each other enough as a parent. In order to be able to reflect and connect, parents need to accept that tragedy is a fact of life and to control their feelings. We see exactly the opposite in parents who are caught up in a high-conflict divorce. The very presence and behaviour of the other arouses intense emotional reactions, causing stress to increase. This may have to do with a battle that has been going on for a long time already – even before the divorce – with both sides unable to accept frustrations and tragedy with the shock and the aftermath of the divorce or with reliving old childhood injuries.

Window of tolerance

Parents feel threatened and get disturbed. They are no longer able to control their emotions or, to quote Siegel (2012), they find themselves outside their window of tolerance; outside a framework in which they can control their feelings. And when tension rises too high and people leave their window of tolerance, they launch into a "survival mode". They start to fight, flight or freeze (FFF). More primitive parts of the brain connected with survival are activated. This is also known as the reptile brain. If the reaction is to fight or to flight, the body is in an active state to escape danger (hyperarousal). If, on the other hand, the reaction is to freeze, the body is in a passive state, which is referred to as hypo-arousal. In both situations, surviving in the here and now is key. There will be limited awareness – a kind of tunnel vision. People will lose contact with reality and conflicts will escalate quickly.

Hostile thoughts (attributions) and feelings

Cognitive factors play an important part in understanding these destructive processes. First, the most important dimensions are causal attributions, defined as the explanation a parent gives for an event or behaviour, and second, responsibility attributions, defined as the extent to which parents hold each other responsible for events (Bradbury & Fincham, 1992).

In systemic therapy, this is known as an interpunction problem. People create order out of the endless flow of information that life brings.

Punctuation is one of the ways to create order. With punctuation, some starting point is considered the reason for the subsequent behaviour. This is how people apply linear sequences to circular connections. The wife says that she has to do the talking because her husband never opens his mouth. The husband, on the other hand, claims that he has to shut his mouth because his wife always does the talking. Both put the blame for their behaviour on the other. And once this order has been created, it will be the framework for ordering new information so that the punctuation will be confirmed, time after time. Information that does not tally with the assumption – with the punctuation – is ignored, and information that confirms the assumption is taken to be true.

In this way, fights can ignite quickly in human relationships. Different punctuations or different assumptions of cause-effect sequences, which are taken to be true, may lead to endless disputes (Savenije, van Lawick & Reijmers, 2014). Parents suffering from a hostile conflict often make attributions (punctuations) about negative events which emphasize the damage and impact of the event and they place the responsibility with the behaviour of the other person. Here, the earlier-mentioned demonizing is at play. They see the other person's behaviour as the cause of the problems, as something stable and unchangeable. They see it as something typical and something that affects many aspects of the relationship and their lives.

Tension mounting up in children, for instance during the handover, is blamed by the parent on the other parent: "My child is always stressed out when she goes to the other. When she is with me, she is herself. It must be an awful place there" or "my child is so stressed out when she returns from the other, that it must be awful there. It takes one or two days for my child to be herself again".

According to scientific literature, these kinds of attributions and punctuations (internal, global, stable) of negative behaviour add to parental conflicts (Bradbury & Fincham, 1992), but the extent to which a parent interprets the other parent's behaviour as malicious, egocentric and objectionable also adds to the intensity and frequency of parental conflicts (Bradbury & Fincham, 1992).

Resentment, anger, distrust

In addition to the cognitive, hostile attributions and punctuation problems, conflicts between partners are also associated with strong negative emotions and defensive reactions such as resentment, anger, distrust, pain and bitterness (Johnston, 1994; Wallerstein, 1986). It is very likely that these emotional reactions will further feed violent and bitter conflicts. This is how distrust of the other parent's ability to take good care of the children adds to more serious conflicts, less cooperation and a lower co-parenting quality (Maccoby & Mnookin, 1992).

Triggers and maintaining factors

Painful and shocking events during or before the relationship with the other parent, and at the time of the divorce and afterwards, often affect the ability to control emotions. The framework within which emotions can still be controlled – the window of tolerance – gets smaller. A parent will easily be hurt by the other parent.

The quick escalation can be explained by means of the information processing model, described by Lang (1985), which explains how meaningful experiences are stored in the memory. Lang starts with the idea that an emotion is made up of different coding. First, the stimulus information: this is the information about an event that has been received through the senses. For instance, information received by the mother via a WhatsApp message: "Could you bring the children earlier today? There is a soccer match they want to go to". Connected to the stimulus information is the level of the meaning information: the meaning people give to the stimulus information. Often, that is the emotional meaning that the parent gives to the message: "There we go again. I am not being taken seriously as a mother". Second, the response: how is the reaction to the stimulus and meaning information. The response has three elements:

- the verbal reaction;
- the autonomous reactions, like sweating, raised heartbeat, and so on;
- the motor reaction, including fight, flight or freeze.

The mother reacts by returning a message: "No, I can't". That is, of course, stimulus information which evokes meaning and responses in the father. The mother feels the stress rising in her body and sits on the couch for an hour, dismayed by the response to the WhatsApp message.

The stronger the associations, the sooner the entire memory network is activated. If events match the various stored representations, an entire network may be activated which evokes the same emotion time and again. Part of the memory (a stimulus, response or meaning representation of the memory) is activated by something in the present, and then the entire network of memories about information, meaning and action is activated. The other one is seen as the perpetrator, as someone who represents danger, including for the child. This results in polarizing and demonizing thoughts: everything or nothing, black or white, perpetrator (the other) or victim (I and the children).

Parents may have negative attributions about the behaviour of the other, but also about themselves. These negative basic thoughts about oneself ("I am a bad mother", "I will be deserted again anyway", "I am a nobody", "I never do things right") are formed in childhood in interactions with important caretakers. This is described in virtually all psychological theories. In attachment theory, this is referred to as "the internal working models" which a child develops about itself in relation to others through experiences with attachment figures (Fonagy, Gergeley & Jurist, 2002).

In scheme theory, they call it "schemes" which children develop and which they use to face up to the world (Vreeswijk, Broersen & Nadort, 2008). In Transactional Analysis (TA) and also in family therapy, this is referred to as "scripts" which constantly repeat themselves (Berne, 1964; Byng-Hall, 1985). It all boils down to the same thing. Children form an image of themselves through interactions with important caretakers or attachment figures: you matter, you are worth a lot, you are loved, you deserve a hug, I am there if you need me and so on. Or, on the contrary: sometimes I am there for you, sometimes I'm not; you are difficult and annoying; you are not okay; you are no good; and so on. If these messages are repeated over and over again, the child will form an image of itself, of the outside world, and of interactions with others which match these messages and affects life.

Usually, children are handed a multitude of images of which the positive images prevail, resulting in a varied self-image. This varied self-image enables people to be flexible with themselves, relations and the outside world. But when scripts are rigid and are repeated over and over again, regularly or in an unpredictable way, this will result in rigid expectations in children, adolescents and, later, adults. In the beginning of a relationship, when in love, something seems to change: "This person does love me, he/she protects me, accepts me as I am, really is there for me and thinks I am okay". The other scripts remain active in the background, but are less dominant. If, however, the old script is activated by painful relational experiences and frustrations, the script can come to the fore again and the old working model may start to colour interactions again. "You see, I will be deserted anyway", "I am not okay", "I never do things right" and so on. The pain and anger are targeted at the person itself and at the person who causes the wounds to be re-opened.

Vulnerability cycle

Scheinkman and Dekoven Fishbane (2004) propose the concept of the vulnerability cycle. The vulnerability of one person, for instance the fear and expectation of being deserted, triggers a survival strategy to feel less pain, for instance control and pursue. This may precisely affect the vulnerability of the wife. She feels small and overwhelmed, and as a survival strategy she will withdraw. This withdrawal affects the very vulnerability of the husband, who will feel deserted and will start to control even more. This is how conflicts often escalate via vulnerabilities. We see this a lot in high-conflict divorces. And other people are often drawn into this painful battle: the social network will play a part in the battle and add to it.

2.2.2 Active involvement of the network

It is a known fact among professionals that the structure and opinions of the social network are especially impactful on the decision-making process of parents who have separated. Social support from the network is one of the key factors that help people cope with stressful life events and divorce (Cohen & Wills, 1985; Lazarus & Folkman, 1984). The social network contributes to the well-being of the individual ex-partner, but the opinions of the social network may also impede efforts of divorced parents to reconcile and negotiate with each other. Although social network partners are very important during the course of a divorce, this has received little attention so far. Not in scientific literature, neither in clinical practice. That is why we only know a little about who the important social network partners of the divorce partners are and what their effect is on the process; how they add to conflicts and negotiations, or rather how they help find the solution to the interparental conflicts.

To give an example, Sally can boost the self-confidence of her best friend who is in a divorce by saying, "You deserve much better, he is a loser". But, at the same time, she can feed the negative image that her friend has of her ex-partner by saying this and so add to the destructive conflicts and fights. Lawyers are paid to "win", to get the most out of it for their client. It is in their interest to choose the side of their client and to find proof with which they can floor the other party. This does not, to put it mildly, promote cooperative co-parenting.

In scientific literature, there is little information to be found about the structure and opinions of the social network. From clinical experience, however, we know that the influence of the social network is big. Literature suggests that experiencing rejection and stigma from the social network can lead to social withdrawal and more distress after stressful life events (Steuber & Solomon, 2011). It is our experience that both polarizing and stigmatizing reactions from the social network have a negative effect on the post-divorce parental adjustment.

2.2.3 *Arguing about the divorce story and about goals*

Parents who are caught up in a high-conflict divorce usually argue about the divorce story. They have different interests and/or ascribe interests to one another. They strive for different goals for themselves and for the children and/or in parenting. All the arguing and stress about these differences lead to confusion in the children.

For identity development it is important that children have a coherent life story, which is propagated and confirmed by important others (Olthof, 2012). Families involved in a high-conflict divorce often don't have a coherent narrative about the reasons why parents separated and about the extent to which each parent contributed to the divorce. The story about the how and why of the divorce has never come to an end and that is why lives come to a standstill. This creates inner turmoil in all family members, but especially in the children.

Mother is, for instance, convinced that the divorce was started because father fell in love with the neighbour and that everything had been fine before that; that they had been all right together, and that the last holidays with the children had been really nice. Father, however, has a completely different story. He says that their relationship had already long been dead, that he has no good memories at all of their last holidays and that he felt alienated from her. It had all ended already and that it was only after that he had been able to fall in love with someone else, and that the two things are not connected. That he would have left, too, if he hadn't fallen in love. Others start to meddle. Her parents support her in her story and say that they had noticed before how the neighbour had been making a pass at their son-in-law. His parents, on the other hand, support his story, or are angry at him and also support the story of their beloved daughter-in-law. The father will perhaps opt for the safe haven of the new in-laws who receive him with open arms and unconditionally believe his version of the divorce story. In this way, relatives, friends and later also social workers and lawyers all play a role and usually strengthen one of the voices.

Parents will not necessarily and literally tell these stories to their children, but the children hear fragments of stories, via parents and via others, and they read e-mails. They catch fragments of telephone conversations and they feel the agitation and the tension about the story and the mutual distrust in particular. It will raise questions in the children's minds about the reliability of parents. Who speaks the truth and who do I look like? This creates a lot of confusion. Children also carry the sense of unease caused by the confusion with them and this affects their well-being as well as the perception and the shaping of their identity.

Goals, wishes, expectations

A conflict of interests which the ex-partners experience (e.g. he only thinks of himself, while I think of the children) about goals, wishes and expectations (e.g. I try to be flexible, while she wants me to stick to the agreements), as well as an obstacle to effective behaviour they experience (e.g. each time I want to talk to him, he gets aggressive and does not listen) further aggravate conflicts between (ex-)partners (Fincham & Beach, 1999).

Experiencing conflicting goals in intimate relationships will reduce satisfaction with the relationship as well as the subjective well-being. These people are less satisfied with life, they have less positive and more negative feelings (Gere & Schimmack, 2013). Take, for instance, a mother who has made it her aim to be a good, caring parent and therefore wants to spend a lot of time with the children and wants to see them during the weekend to be able to engage with them. And a father who has made it his aim to release the children from their mother's smothering behaviour and therefore wants the children to stay with him as often as possible. In such a situation it is very difficult for parents to solve the conflict between these two goals.

Another thing is that many parents experience inequality in a high-conflict divorce. They feel that they are being treated unfairly and unequally by the other parent and, for that reason alone, they are not able to come to an agreement.

In high-conflict divorces it is often about a "fair" share of time with the children, about finances, housing and so on. It seems that conflicts aggravate when parents experience unfairness and inequality in the relationship with the other parent about these matters.

- People who feel slighted in terms of tangible and intangible resources which they are entitled to (such as money, housing, emotional investment, time, efforts) experience pain and feel they are being treated unfairly (Greenstein, 2009). One parent weighs his/her costs against those of the other, concludes that his/her costs are higher and then feels slighted.

- People who feel slighted are motivated to put in a lot of effort to restore the balance and equality in the relationship (Kluwer, Heesink & van de Vliert, 2002).
- Divorces happen more often when a partner (usually the wife) feels less happy than the other partner (usually the husband) (Guven, Senik & Stichnoth, 2012).

These findings not only suggest that experiences of inequality impede post-divorce adjustment, but also that they motivate parents to strike back; to fight and to seek for means to enforce a new balance and equality, such as taking revenge and impeding the partner's goals.

Both parents often feel that they are making too many concessions already, or that the other thinks too negatively about him or her. This further reduces the chance that the conflict will be settled in a constructive way. This battle to achieve equality stands in the way of combining and integrating different goals and wishes. As parents experience that the conflicts exhaust all energy and resources, thus impeding recovery and personal growth, the parental conflict may expand to include other goals. So, especially in high-conflict divorces, which are full of opposite goals, parents must find ways to accommodate their goal-oriented behaviour to one another, often on a daily basis.

The solution to such conflicting goals lies either in pursuing self-interest (pursuing the own goal) or in meeting the other's interest (Rusbult & Van Lange, 2003). In high-conflict divorces, that choice is complicated by the fact that parents often think that they have the child's goal in mind. They assume that the child thinks and feels like they do. Parents also often make the mistake of thinking that the other parent will hurt the child in the same way as he/she hurt her/himself. This, however, does not need to be the case at all. As a parent, parents can sometimes get the best out of themselves. This may be very different from how they are as a partner.

In order to get out of conflicts about goals and interests, parents therefore have to be able to give due weight to the interest of the other parent and that of the children, and sometimes even put that interest before their own (Rusbult & Van Lange, 2003).

This makes identifying common goals and increasing the ability to constructively resolve conflicts one of the biggest challenges in high-conflict divorces. Defining concrete goals gives parents room to think about ways to realize these goals. It helps them to achieve the goal (Gollwitzer & Brandstatter, 1997). Goals may be about the house and living, about parenting, dividing means and money, and following parenting styles.

An important goal is the new parenting style: parallel solo parenthood (Cottyn, 2009) or, rather, a cooperative parenting team. Cottyn explains the divorce battle by pointing at the confusion about finding a new parenting organization. She calls it a complex transition. She believes that both parents feel responsible, but that the battle about the parenting organization dominates everything. She warns of the illusion of social workers that they can help all divorced parents in forming a good parenting team that is able to cooperate without arguing. If parents have already been arguing for a long time, this is an over-romantic ideal. Sometimes, taking some distance and stopping the interfering in each other's business is exactly what it takes to smooth the waters for the children.

With parallel solo parenthood, parents each focus on their own situation with the children and try to do their very best in their own house. They let go of each other and do not (or no longer) interfere in the other parent's affairs. This will stop the demonizing, and allows for more peace and for an environment of trust for the children. There is minimal contact between the parents. This may be a temporary phase or it may take longer. Later on, parents may start to form a cooperative and connected team and visit each other again. This, however, is only possible if the tension has eased and confidence has increased.

2.2.4 Children falling off the radar

It is striking to see that children are often the topic of conversation where, in reality, they often fall off the radar. Parents, grandparents, the wider network and social workers all talk about the children, but hardly anyone really asks the children how they are doing, what they feel and what they need. On the contrary, discussions about the children become part of the battle.

In practice, professionals see that parents in a high-conflict divorce often claim that they fight "to protect the children" or "for the sake of the children". Parents are convinced that the other parent does not possess the right parenting skills and they think that they themselves are the better parent (Johnston, 1994). Sometimes, one parent accuses the other of neglecting or abusing the children. Both parents view themselves as the sole representative of the child's interests. They see themselves as the gatekeeper of the child's safety and well-being. Parents think that they have right on their side because they represent the interest of their child: they think they fight the battle for their children instead of for themselves. But in reality, the very needs and interest of the child are overlooked due to the bitter fights and battle between the parents. The very

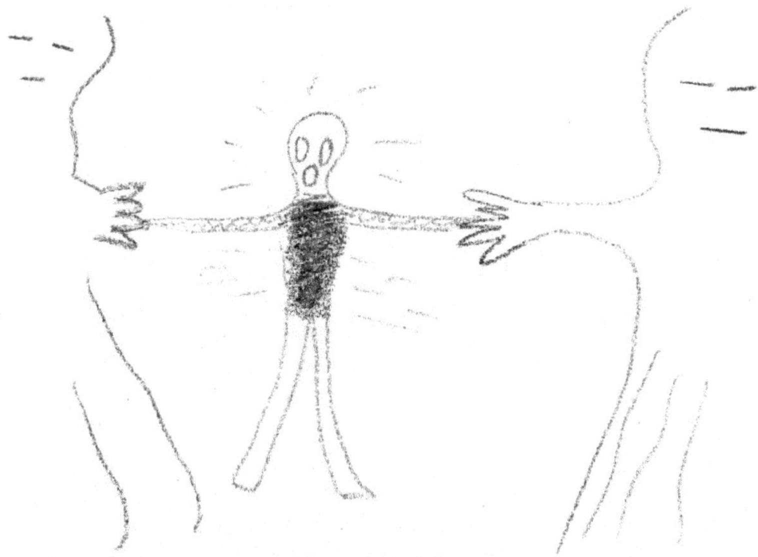

Figure 2.1 Child off the radar

battle hampers effective parenting (Fotheringham, Dunbar & Hensley, 2013). A study shows that this is an important theme in battles between high-conflict divorced (HCD) parents: concerns about the child's safety and well-being when they are left in the care of the other parent. This especially seems to be the case when the children are still very young (Cashmore & Parkinson, 2011).

There are indications that these types of feelings and thoughts of superiority exactly, and the fact that a parent thinks that he or she represents the interest of the child better than the other parent, aggravate the fights and communication between parents. The idea that someone is acting in the interest of someone else leads to more intense conflicts, less forgivingness and less cooperation in negotiations (Wildschut et al., 2003).

An example of what that may lead to is parental alienation syndrome.

Parental alienation syndrome

In the US, parental alienation syndrome (PAS) was first defined by Gardner (1998) as "a disorder that arises primarily in the context of child custody disputes". PAS is manifested by a campaign of denigration of one parent and the child against the other parent. A campaign with no valid motive and in which children lack ambivalent feelings: one parent is good and the other is bad. The children do not feel guilty about their behaviour towards the rejected parent. Research in the US and in the Netherlands shows that parental alienation, or parental rejection, occurs in approximately ten per cent of divorce children. The child usually targets the father, as the child lives with the mother more often. Johnston (2006) concludes that alienated children run a significantly higher risk of an adverse development, such as depression, low self-esteem and high drug and alcohol use. The greater the measure of parental alienation, the higher the measure of anxiety, depression and aggression in children. Parental alienation is typically experienced negatively by the alienated parent, usually the father.

In the context of the parental alienation syndrome, one parent feels superior because he or she follows the child in rejecting the other parent. The other parent feels superior as he or she points out the harmful effects of parental alienation for the child. Not surprisingly, the father's movement often points out the damaging effects of parental alienation and puts the blame on the mother (Zander, 2011). The battle between parents intensifies and leads to further polarization and to a perpetrator-victim dynamic. This dynamic plays a role in the family, the social network and in society. An important point of criticism made by Kelly and Johnston (2001) is that attention is focussed too much on the "programming parent" as the source of evil. The discussion about this syndrome, which is attributed to children, particularly concerns the adults – the parents (Bernet et al., 2010).

We would like to add our reflections to these views. In our view, it is about an impaired parent-child relationship. These children grow up in an environment where nearly everyone polarizes, thinks black-and-white, demonizes and does not tolerate ambivalence. Parents often express unreasonably negative feelings and opinions about the other parent, which are typically out of proportion to actual experiences. Not surprisingly, children growing up in a dependent relationship adopt the demonizing thoughts and remarks of the parent they spend most of the time with, especially since the network of this parent shares these beliefs.

We therefore wonder why it is that the children are burdened with the diagnosis of parental alienation or parental rejection syndrome. It is our belief that the child itself is falling off the radar. We cannot expect children to keep on thinking for themselves, to stay unbiased and to be able to live in two "truths" when the adults around them are not able to do so. Another factor is that children, to survive (biologically), depend on the parent they live with. Children, of all people, cannot continue to live in two truths, and it is an extreme survival mechanism to side with one of the truths. The adults around them are doing the same thing. We think that on this point, too, parents should be at the heart of the treatment.

In high-conflict divorces, it is the parents who suffer from mutual parental alienation or parent rejection syndrome. The parents alienate themselves from each other – from the other parent with whom they had a child. They reject and demonize the other parent. The child merely copies that behaviour as part of a survival mechanism. We think that, in general, it is best for the children to have contact with and to spend time with both parents, unless one of the parents evidently does not function properly. Parents who come to us have already seen several social workers, and if there were concerns about functioning, these have already been investigated. The parents who come to see us are not perfect, but they can function well enough. For instance, by allowing the child to see both parents.

This is the vision behind the No Kids in the Middle programme. We have often experienced that children can have contact with both parents again if the parents reconcile in some way; if they no longer continuously run each other down and if they stop rejecting or alienating themselves from the other parent. A daughter recently put it like this in a family meeting: "If you two start treating each other normally again, I don't mind to be with you, mum". In general, children are very able to make it clear how much they suffer from parents abusing each other and running each other down.

Marsha Pinedo (www.villapinedo.nl) has done pioneering work in The Netherlands. She set up an organization for and by children of divorced parents. The webpage of Villa Pinedo contains a few open letters from children. Time and again, children appear to not really be heard and seen in the divorce process of their parents. If children are seen and heard, they will be all right again as time goes by after the divorce. That is why Marsha Pinedo wrote a book for parents getting a divorce with accompanying online training dealing with all the important steps and how they may go through all the changes with the child in mind (Pinedo & Vollinga, 2013).

Divorced parents who are caught up in conflicts have often lost this perspective along the way. They use the child and its experiences, by their own definitions, in their fight against the other, and in the process it is the child who falls off the radar.

2.2.5 Powerlessness

Another characteristic of high-conflict divorces is the huge sense of powerlessness that the parties involved in the divorce feel. Both the parents themselves, the children and the network often experience a great sense of powerlessness. They have done a lot to improve the situation, but because of the persistent battle, they are often unable to bring about a structural change. Parents continue to force the other to change. The network is in it, too. Professionals try to stop the battle and to bring parents to reason.

Classification

If all efforts end in failure, people usually start to classify the problem. Classifying and diagnosing the other parent as mentally disturbed is especially quite common. The rationale behind this seems to be that "If all my efforts to improve the situation end in failure, the other parent surely must be disturbed".

The intense emotional reactions in the battle often lead to the assumption that the person in question is suffering from borderline personality disorder. This is not so surprising because a borderline personality disorder is characterized by black-and-white thinking, frenetically trying to prevent being deserted, a negative self-image, impulsive behaviour and inadequate anger (DSM-IV). All of these factors are common in high-conflict divorces.

Pedagogical differences – one parent is a little messier and easier, and the other is a bit more rigid – are often linked to psychopathology, more specifically to attention deficit disorders (ADD or ADHD) or compulsive disorders (OCD). Part of this behaviour can be connected with survival strategies. Parents who, for instance, try to stay away from the battle by increasingly avoiding each other can be labelled "autistic" or "narcissist".

Professionals, too, often assume that psychopathology is involved; for instance, narcissism. People with a high score of narcissism show little empathy (Decety & Jackson, 2004), are often aggressive when they feel threatened (Bushman & Baumeister, 1998), are less forgiving and more resentful (Exline et al., 2004), and, to conclude, focus more on their own interest than on that of the partner when communicating with their partner (Vangelisti, Knapp & Daly, 1990).

Each one of these characteristics can easily be linked to parents in a divorce battle. Parents are often fully convinced of the accuracy of the diagnosis of psychopathology in the other parent: "I checked it on the internet, and it all fits. It's perfectly clear". Borderline personality problems and psychopathy are also often mentioned as classifications.

In the No Kids in the Middle programme, we take the same position as we do with children who are reported with numerous symptoms. The stress of the divorce battle makes people vulnerable, anxious and rigid in their reactions. It is only when people experience more safety and less stress that it is possible to see where there are still concerns and where additional help and treatment is needed. We do not challenge diagnoses but continue to focus on reducing stress and creating a safer environment in which children can grow up well, and that also works out well for parents and their networks. Usually, symptoms will decrease in the process.

In that respect, we consider classifying and diagnosing as a form of demonizing. The powerlessness makes people look for something outside themselves – a demon. A psychiatric disorder suits this purpose very well. There is a cause, the cause lies in the other, the other should have him/herself treated and then things may get better. And this is how powerlessness and reacting to powerlessness are also connected with the first characteristic: demonization.

2.2.6 *Stagnated transition*

A last characteristic is that parents in a high-conflict divorce have not made the transition from being together to separating and letting go. They are not really separated, but continue to be involved with each other. They remain stuck in the phase between separating and landing in a new life where they are no longer involved with their ex-partner like they used to be. Sometimes, parents only had been in a very short relationship, but they continue to be involved with the ex-partner because of the continuous conflicts and, as a result, they do not let go of each other. The fact that they remain stuck in an intermediate stage is very aggravating. Life freezes. Parents feel like they cannot move on with their lives.

This can be compared to migration. Migrants must let go of their old country, including their old house, their own language and culture. They enter a transition phase, the liminal stage. This phase starts with the (refugee) trip to the country of destination and lasts until the migrant receives a residence permit, gets the opportunity to work and can focus on integration into the new life. (Rhmaty, 2011). It is a known fact that most problems and symptoms occur in the liminal stage, which has to do with uncertainty. Migrants in refugee camps are in the liminal stage. Many of them are depressed, aggressive, violent, anxious and even psychotic. There will be rest when they have a house and can integrate. They can focus on a new life with work and perhaps a relationship or a family. Usually, this rest makes the serious symptoms disappear.

A divorce is also a transition with a liminal stage. Usually, the conflicts come to rest in the course of the year after the divorce. Parents in a high-conflict divorce remain stuck in the intermediate stage, the liminal stage, sometimes for as long as ten years and, in exceptional cases, forever. Not only the parents, but also the children and the people around them, remain stuck in this stage. To help them make the transition, parents need to learn to let go. Let go of the illusion of control and start focussing on themselves and their own life. If they manage to do so, they will have more energy and they will be available for their children again. The energy leak of the high-conflict divorce, which literally makes many people ill, will be stopped when they make the transition to real separation and can integrate into a new life.

2.3 Interventions

Professionals working with families in a high-conflict divorce often get tired and frustrated. They struggle with several dilemmas. Meanwhile, however, they must try to offer the proper support, care, information and help to parents who are caught up in bitter conflicts, and to their children suffering from that. Often, there is not enough focus on the well-being of the children. That is why interventions which put the child's well-being first are badly needed when it comes to these problems.

As far as we know, no proven and effective intervention has been developed so far, at home or abroad, for these parents and children. Several descriptive articles have been written about interventions for these families, but they have not been scientifically tested for efficacy (Lebow & Rekart, 2007; Spillane-Grieco, 2000).

Note

1 Catrin Finkenauer supported us by conducting a literature search. Her summary helped us writing this part and forms the basis for the development of No Kids in the Middle.

Chapter 3

Scientific research

3.1 Introduction

No Kids in the Middle is an intervention developed from practice. In the clinical setting we offered treatments to families caught up in a conflict divorce which were not effective enough. We were not able to come to grips with the destructive interparental conflicts, and we could not relieve the pain in the children. At the same time, we were offering group treatments for other types of family problems at the Lorentzhuis (Centre for systemic therapy, training and consultation) and the KJTC (Children's Trauma Centre), and these group treatments were found to be effective. That is why we developed a group treatment for the families.

We then went on to give the treatment a scientific basis and started to formulate research questions. We did so in consultation with other therapists, scientific researchers and with the parents.

Until recently, psychotherapeutic treatments were considered effective, in particular if research had been done with a randomized controlled trial (RCT). This means that a group receiving treatment is compared to a group not receiving treatment (the control group). Evidence-based working means that, preferably, treatments are given which are "proven effective" after multiple RCTs. It is a top-down approach: practice implements what science claims to be effective. Fortunately, practice-based evidence is getting more and more recognition these days. It is a bottom-up approach, from practice: the therapist makes implicit practical knowledge explicit. He or she evaluates this knowledge with clients, incorporating it into the treatment. In doing so, practical knowledge can lead and add to theoretical knowledge.

That is what we have done. First, we summarized the answers to the research questions in this chapter. Then, we discussed the study results and its implication for the intervention with the parents in the groups in treatment at the time. We talked about the results of the children's experiences as well as the implication for the intervention with a group of adolescents with high-conflict divorced parents. Finally, we discussed the study results and the reflections of the adolescents with various providers of the No Kids in the Middle programme. The opinions of researchers, parents, adolescents and providers have been incorporated into the intervention, as described in Part 2 of this book, "Practice".

Of course, we are already busy formulating new research questions together with researchers, providers, parents and adolescents. In this way, we ensure the continuous interplay of practice and science.

3.2 Study in the Dutch language area

From April 2014 to July 2016, the Academic Collaborative Centre Child Abuse (Academische Werkplaats aanpak Kindermishandeling (AWK) conducted a scientific study of parents and children taking part in the No Kids in the Middle programme in the Netherlands and Belgium. The AWK is a cooperative of the VU University Amsterdam and the KJTC (Children's Trauma Centre). The study was carried out by Prof Dr. C. Finkenauer, Dr. Kim Schoemaker, Annelies de Kruijf MA and Dr. Margreet Visser. Justine van Lawick and various other colleagues from the Lorentzhuis, the KJTC and the VU University were involved in the study design. In total, 17 different institutions throughout the Netherlands and Belgium took part in the study, some with more than one group. A total of 27 groups were included.

Parents are usually referred to the No Kids in the Middle programme via child protection services or by judges. The referrers are concerned about the development of the children, as they are caught between the parents. Parents can register themselves, too. They fill out an online questionnaire before the start of No Kids in the Middle (pre measure) and afterwards (post measure). Six months after the intervention, parents receive a request by email to fill out a short follow-up questionnaire.

Children between the ages of six to 18 can participate in the study, for which both custodial parents must give informed consent. To make sure that children are not put under pressure or feel forced to give certain answers, the children fill out the questionnaire during the first and the last group session of No Kids in the Middle. They can do so on paper or via a link on the computer or iPad. There are three different versions available of the questionnaire, and they are linked to the child's age.

This study comprehensively deals with what children and parents go through, feel and think in a conflict divorce. We look, for instance, at what problems children do and do not experience, and we ask them who they turn to for support. We try to find out how parents think about each other and how they adjust to the divorce.

The study focusses on the following questions:

1. Who are the parents and the children taking part in No Kids in the Middle?
2. How do the children experience the conflicts and the divorce?
3. What changes in behaviour and feelings are observed in parents and children after participating in the No Kids in the Middle intervention?
4. What is the link between the changes in the parents and those in the children?
5. What is the role of forgiving and of the social network in parental conflicts?
6. What is the role of trust and of interpersonal processes in parental conflicts?

3.2.1 Research question 1: Description of the study population

The study focussed on the question: Who are the HCD parents and their children? Finkenauer et al. (2017) answered this question. A summary of the article in question follows.

The population of the study consisted of 165 divorced parents, of whom there were 83 fathers and 82 mothers. The age of the parents ranged between 26 and 66 years old. Fathers had a mean age of 43.5 and mothers had a mean age of 41. The group of parents appeared to be diverse, especially in terms of type and duration of the relationship prior to the divorce. Some parents did not have a relationship; others had been together for a long time (up to 27 years). The parents were relatively highly educated.

On average, the parents have two children. Almost one-third have one child, and that is a high percentage compared to the Dutch average of ten per cent. The large majority of divorced parents have joint custody and a new partner. Of the parents with a new relationship, one-third have a child with the new partner.

Most of the communication between parents is in writing, via email or WhatsApp. Three-quarters of the parents indicate that they often communicate in this way. Half of the parents only communicate in writing. We asked parents about their most important reasons to go for a divorce. On average, they mention three different reasons. The two most important are too many conflicts and bad communication (both 56%). It is remarkable to find that both parents do not always give the same answers when it comes to their child(ren), especially when it comes to care for the children and the place where they live.

There were 142 children who took part in the study, 75 of whom were boys and 67 of whom were girls. The children ranged between the ages of six and 18, with a mean age of ten years. Almost two-thirds of the children receive care.

The time span after the divorce until the start of No Kids in the Middle varies considerably, from zero to 12 years, with a mean duration of 4.5 years. It implies that children are often exposed to conflicts and arguments between parents for years. The divorce often has serious consequences for the income, which will decrease for the average parent, especially for women.

3.2.2 Research question 2: How do children experience the conflicts and the divorce?

The results of this study are described in the report of Schoemaker et al., 2017. The children clearly describe how they experience the situation of the conflicts and the divorce. They find it particularly hard to deal with:

- changing houses;
- parents having different rules;
- their belongings being in the other house;
- the feeling that they have to choose between father and mother and;
- parents speaking ill of each other.

Research has shown that almost all children of divorced parents suffer from these issues. In "normal" divorces, children are perfectly able to deal with them after an average of one year (Spruijt & Kormos, 2014). Children of parents in a conflict divorce continue to struggle with these issues for as long as their parents have been separated (on average 4.5 years). These children indicate that parents do not jointly decide on these issues, they do not agree and continue to fight. It seems as if the transition from a family living together to a family of parents living apart is not made; as if parents remain caught in the transition phase with the corresponding burden for the children. See also section 2.2.6.

The interspace

We refer to "interspace" as the relational space in which parents need to work together. In this space, they have to organize how the child will go from one parent to the other and on which days and at what times, how birthdays and holidays are celebrated and where, how holidays are split up and organized, how finances are managed and who buys the coats and shoes, what will be for dinner and so on. This is where the children experience tension and conflicts – where they are torn and feel caught in the middle.

Many children indicate that they worry about their family and that, especially at home with their parents, they suffer from the divorce. A majority of the older children (12 years old and up) say that they suffer from the divorce while learning in the classroom. One-third of the children indicate that they suffer from the divorce during other activities, and one-quarter of the children have trouble coping with the arguments between their parents in friendships and when at their grandparents'. It is a good sign that a majority of the children suffer less from the divorce when they are busy doing other activities. Divorce-related difficulties therefore seem to be tied to the context. Our study, however, does not provide insight into how children feel when parents meet each other at, for instance, parents' evenings, sporting events, school trips or performances. In clinical practice, we often hear that children find it hard to deal with these situations.

The majority of the children say that they can turn to their mother (63%) with their worries; a minority (40%) say that they can turn to their father. Their best friends, brothers or sisters are also often mentioned as confidential advisers. It is remarkable to find that more than one-third of the children say that they share their worries with their teacher. This underlines the important part that school plays for children of divorced parents.

3.2.3 Research question 3: Change study

The results of this study are described in the report of Schoemaker et al., 2017. For research question 3, we have mapped the changes in parents and children by comparing pre and post measures. A total of 110 parents have completed both the pre and post measures. That is 67 per cent of the 165 parents who completed the pre measure. To test whether a change can be seen in time, a change between men and women, and a difference in change between men and women, the data have been analyzed with a repeated-measures analysis of variance (ANOVA), with time (pre and post measures) as the within-subject factor and gender as the between-subject factor. A p-value smaller than 0.05 usually indicates a significant (meaningful) change or effect. Since many different tests have been conducted, we used a Bonferroni correction for the number of tests. We speak of a significant change or effect only if revealed after the

Bonferroni correction. In the analyses, we did not, as a rule, find a difference between men and women in the extent of change.

3.2.3.1 Change in parents

Parents report, in particular, change in behaviour; as time goes by, there will be less conflicts. Parents report that these conflicts are more constructive and less serious after the No Kids in the Middle intervention. This is what the children report, too.

Changes which parents report seem to be connected, in particular, with positive processes:

- Parents forgive each other more easily.
- They find it easier to accept the divorce.
- We also find a tendency for parents to trust each other a little more.

At the same time, we see no or hardly any change in especially negative processes. The parents:

- think as badly about the ex-partner as before;
- put the blame for the conflicts on the other one as often as before;
- feel the same about the ex-partner.

We asked parents about their relationship with their children. We do not find any changes here. Parents think that they have a good relationship with their children and that they are available. Parents also have the impression that children think they matter to their parents. The good relationship that most parents mention in the pre measure may be the reason for the fact that parents do not experience any change. It is also possible that parents find it difficult to put themselves in their children's shoes. Maybe they do not really know what their children feel for the parents and what they feel when they are with both parents.

Dr. Aurelie Lange, senior researcher at mental healthcare centre de Viersprong, is currently analyzing the data of the follow-up measure (a questionnaire filled out by the parents four to six months after the intervention). She compares the results with a reference group of "normal" divorces.

3.2.3.2 Change in children

The study shows a very varied pattern in children. On the one hand, children indicate that they are doing fine: about the past week, they say that they feel well and that they are happy with their lives. Adolescents indicate that they feel they belong somewhere. They have self-confidence, are in control of their lives and think life is meaningful. Adolescent girls score worse than boys on this point. We find that No Kids in the Middle does not change this. After the intervention, they are still doing fine. This outcome is different from what we had expected.

On the other hand, children indicate that they can experience the divorce as traumatic. Half of the children in our study score so high on trauma complaints that they run a high risk of getting post-traumatic stress disorder (PTSD). After No Kids in the Middle, the children score lower on trauma complaints, but the improvement is not significant.

Children explain that they have a good relationship with both their father and mother and that they matter. We asked children to judge their mother and father separately. We think that children have a good relationship with each individual parent, but that in the very interspace described previously, tension and stress arise in the children's lives. Instances of this include when parents refuse to bring things they forgot, or when one parent talks badly about the other. In this interspace, children are at risk of being traumatized. The question is also if children feel seen when they talk about the other house or the other parent or stepparent (see also section 3.4.4, Compartmentalization).

We have also considered if differences between children can be explained by age or gender. That does not appear from the results. The differences may possibly depend on other factors, such as the severity of the parental conflicts or the period of time the parents have already been separated. Van der Wal, Finkenauer and Visser (2019) have looked on an individual level at how the seemingly conflicting results of the children (high well-being and a high risk of PTSD) relate to each other. Children who experience the divorce as more traumatic also report a lower level of well-being.

3.2.4 Research question 4: Link between changes in parents and in children

Dr. Aurelie Lange is studying the link between changes in parents and changes in children following intervention. She does so in cooperation with Prof Dr. R.J.H. Scholte and Dr. Margreet Visser. At the time of publication of this book, the articles have not yet been published. After publication, the results will be published online on the website www.kinderenuitdeknel.nl/nokidsinthemiddle.com

3.2.5 Research question 5: Role of forgiving and the social network

Visser et al. (2017) have studied the role of forgiving and the social network in parental conflicts. When parents continue to have conflicts after the divorce and do not solve these conflicts, this may lead to children performing badly. But it is not clear how interparental conflicts are maintained and/or escalate further. We think that the social network plays a part in this.

With research question 5 we examined whether co-parenting conflicts are associated with perceived social network disapproval of the ex-partner, and whether this relation is mediated by parents' tendency to forgive each other. We examined this in a group of "normal" divorces (136 parents) and a group of HCD parents (110 parents). Results show that parents who perceive a more negative attitude towards the other parent have more co-parenting conflicts. We explain this relationship by the tendency to forgive; the more the social network disapproves, the less forgiveness and the more parenting conflicts. This plays a role in both normal and high-conflict divorces.

We also looked at factors other than forgiveness which may mediate the link between the social network and the conflicts:

- the parents' educational level;
- the duration of the relationship of the parents;
- the time elapsed since the divorce; and
- the parents' gender.

We did not find any link with these factors. A unique element of the No Kids in the Middle treatment is its attention on the social network. Despite the fact that the network is explicitly involved in No Kids in the Middle, we have not found any indications of change in the perceived social network disapproval of the ex-partner.

3.2.6 Research question 6: What is the role of trust between parents?

Finkenauer et al. (2018) have examined the role of trust, forgiveness, appreciation, contempt and hostile attributions between parents in conflict. We know that in relationships where people trust each other, there are less conflicts than in relationships where people trust each other less. It is also common knowledge that trust reduces negative processes between people and, on the contrary, allows for positive processes.

We expect that more trust even allows for ex-partners to forgive and appreciate each other, and that more trust reduces contempt and hostile attributions regarding the ex-partner.

We have examined this in a group of 165 ex-partners with children (from 58 couples) who were involved in a conflict divorce. Our hypothesis was confirmed. Ex-partners who have more trust in their ex also have fewer conflicts about parenting, and this is found to be associated with more forgiveness, more appreciation, less contempt and less hostile attributions. So the more Mary trusts Oscar, the more she appreciates him and forgives him, and the fewer conflicts she experiences; and the more she trusts Oscar, the less she despises him and the less she feels he is to blame for the arguments, and the fewer conflicts she experiences.

We also found significant partner effects, which implies that the trust of the ex-partner also influences the level of co-parenting conflicts. In other words, Mary experiences fewer conflicts if Oscar trusts her more. There are no differences in the results between men and women. In terms of the conflict level, there is no link with the duration of the divorce. It is therefore important that therapists focus on the trust level of both ex-partners when designing intervention programmes for ex-partners in a conflict divorce.

3.3 Outline international research

Since 2016, No Kids in the Middle has been implemented in various countries. Currently, a research study is being conducted in Norway and Germany. At the time of the publication of this book, results of two qualitative research studies in Norway and Belgium have been published. An outline is provided in the following sections. The results of international research studies will also be published on the website of No Kids in the Middle.

3.3.1 Norway

In Norway, one group has been evaluated in a qualitative study in which all parents (n=10) were interviewed twice, once right before the start of the programme and once about two months after the last evening of the therapy. The parents were interviewed by people other than the therapists. All interviews were recorded on tape and transcribed before being analyzed.

The parents assess No Kids in the Middle as a good intervention. A large majority also feel that participation has had positive effects on their parenting role and/or on the children's functioning, which has led to better arrangements about parental access, better communication and cooperation with the children, and fewer interparental conflicts. A flexible implementation, where the participants received individual coaching according to their needs and empathic coaching by the therapists, have probably contributed to the positive results.

3.3.2 *Belgium – Leuven*

Researcher Lisa van der Meulen did qualitative research through in-depth interviews with ten Flemish therapists conducting the group intervention programme No Kids in the Middle. In general, therapists are very enthusiastic about the potential and the effects of this new intervention. There is, however, bad policy. Therapists are not allowed enough time for implementation. They also experience a lot of stress and frustration due to overtime, lots of extra work and the difficult target group. Most therapists were able to share these frustrations with a colleague. In this way, the programme also made for a feeling of solidarity between colleagues and organizations. The therapists also felt that the programme had enhanced their personal and professional development. Apart from this learning experience, all therapists considered the supervisions very useful. A positive impact is also seen in the parents and the children, especially in the support that parents and children experience from one another and is frequently mentioned as a strength. Another strength is that children are given a voice through the presentations (Meulen, 2017).

3.4 Conclusions and clinical implications

In this last section, we look back on the many aspects of the study. We also reflect on the implications of the study results for theory and practice when it comes to parents caught up in a high-conflict divorce and their children. We work in a continuous cycle in which clinical practice is fed by results from scientific research, and scientific research builds on questions from clinical practice.

The study is a preliminary indication that the No Kids in the Middle intervention is effective for families caught up in a high-conflict divorce. Both parents and children report a decrease in parental conflicts after the intervention. The measure of demonization of the other parent, however, remains the same after the intervention. On the other hand, parents do forgive each other more after No Kids in the Middle. There is a tendency that they trust the other parent more and accept the divorce better. Qualitative research, together with parents, will help us gain more insight into these sometimes conflicting results.

The intervention takes approximately four to six months. Taking part in No Kids in the Middle certainly impacted the families, but they have no doubt experienced events (for instance holidays, death, birthdays, new partner, births, new job, dismissal, moving house) which have played a role, too. The fact that legal proceedings must be stopped during No Kids in the Middle may also have an effect. That is why we must consider our findings preliminary.

3.4.1 Parental conflicts

Parents mainly report a change in behaviour: eventually there were fewer conflicts and parents indicated that these conflicts were more constructive and less serious after the No Kids in the Middle intervention. This is also what children reported. Different aspects of the intervention may have contributed to this change.

First, it is possible that due to the intervention, parents start to have some contact with each other again – half of the parents never had any personal contact before the start of the intervention – which may have made the conflicts more constructive. Communication by email seems to more easily lead to conflict escalation than face-to-face communication (Friedman & Currall, 2003).

Second, it is possible that specific components in the parent treatment contribute to fewer conflicts. For instance, taking on the perspective of the child or that of the other parent, role play, changing the demonizing story, conflict handling, letting go of the illusion of control and making the transition to real separation.

Third, it is possible that parent-child components of No Kids in the Middle (for instance, confrontation with thoughts and feelings of children about the divorce) make parents realize that children suffer from the conflicts, which will make them increase their efforts to reduce the conflicts. Future research may provide more insight into how the intervention has possibly contributed to a reduction of conflicts, such as by conducting in-depth interviews with parents.

3.4.2 Positive processes between parents

The results also reveal that parents forgive each other more and accept the divorce better after the intervention than before. We also observe a trend that parents start to trust each other more. Specific components of the parent treatment may also have contributed to this, for instance the assignment to mention some positive points of the ex-partner's parenting, the assignment to write a new story about the divorce in which the other parent does not get all the blame and by explaining the concept of forgiving.

These findings underline the importance of positive processes between parents. Today's literature largely ignores such positive processes and focusses almost exclusively on negative processes (conflict, negative emotions, blaming, anger) between parents and the impact of these processes on children. We know surprisingly little about how positive processes like forgiving work, not only in the relationship between parents, but also in the relationship between parents and children.

Also in the clinical practice of No Kids in the Middle, therapists report that parents seem to accept each other's differences more and to find the other parent "good enough" as a parent, even though most parents still don't like the other parent. Research by Gottman (1998) and others (Baumeister et al., 2001; Frederickson, 2009) shows that couples who have three to five times more positive than negative interactions can maintain good relationships for a longer time. In our therapeutic attitude towards parents, we have increasingly emphasized the support of the parents. In Western culture, we tend to address parents sternly and disapprovingly about what they do to their children with their continuous conflicts. We emphasize the positive processes by supporting the parents in letting go, trusting, appreciating and forgiving each other again. And we keep on linking that to the parenting. So, what does it mean for the children when they notice that you trust and appreciate each other again? And how can we, the therapists, help you there?

All sessions of No Kids in the Middle start with a warm-up of parents and children together (see sections 8.2 and 9.2). This allows for a positive and cheerful start for both the parents and the children. Parents, children and therapists do an exercise together for a couple of minutes. This gives parents the opportunity to see that the children can have a good relationship with the other parent, too, and/or that the other parent takes a positive attitude towards the children. In clinical practice, therapists observe that the parents increasingly accept the divorce. See section 2.2.6.

At the same time, we see no or hardly any change in other, especially negative interpersonal processes in the ex-partner and the acceptance of the divorce: neither hostile attributions and negative feelings regarding the partner, nor the appreciation of the ex-partner have changed after the intervention. Negative attribution styles and cognitive distortions in general may be persistent and unwittingly influence the interpretation of situations and behaviour in relationships and contribute to conflict escalation (Fincham & Bradbury, 1987). This may also increase the risk of a return to old conflict styles. In our study, we have also demonstrated the link between negative interpersonal processes, trust and conflicts (see section 3.2.6).

Given these comments, more and sustained research is needed into (the promotion of) positive processes and interactions. Longitudinal and qualitative research especially can help us gain insight into the question whether these changes in parents and children will last and may contribute to the well-being of the parents and children, and to their being able to better adjust to the divorce. Attention for both positive and negative processes is important to better map the processes and to work out how negative processes and their effects can be prevented.

In recent literature, it has been assumed that behaviour is driven by two cognitive systems that are characterized by two qualitatively different thinking processes. The reflective system consists of slow, controlled thinking processes which require effort and are subject to conscious considerations and rules. The impulsive system, on the other hand, is mainly associative and consists of quick and automatic thinking processes (e.g. Friese, Hofmann & Wiers, 2011).

It is possible that the long-lasting interparental battle and conflicts have made the impulsive system become more sensitive to negative stimuli associated with the ex-partner. This is comparable to sensitization in traumatic experiences (Masten & Narayan, 2012). Certain behaviour or character traits of the ex-partner can trigger a negative reaction within a second without one being able to control or steer this. In this case, reflective thinking processes would be more susceptible to change than impulsive thinking processes. Changes like we have found would then be mainly connected with reflective thinking processes which steer this behaviour (e.g. "I need to take trouble to be a good parent for my children by arguing less with my ex") and less with the automatic implicit thinking processes and feelings (e.g. "Pff, there we go again, she gets on my nerves").

During an intervention, ex-partners would then be able to gain more control of reflective thoughts and behaviour that can be consciously steered, but not (yet) of impulsive tendencies, emotions or automatic thoughts. To treat the impulsive system, it would be a better idea to desensitize the negative stimuli associated with the ex-partner. This is what we have done, for instance, during the intake interview by talking about the vulnerability cycle with parents. Parents share how they trigger each other, and the therapists turn this into a connecting story using the vulnerability cycle. Parents can begin to understand how the other parent makes them triggered, how they impulsively react to that and what they can do to get a grip on their own impulses.

It could also help to offer people alternative behaviours to stop unwanted patterns. Research has shown that when people think very deliberately about what they will do in certain situations, chances increase that, in these situations, they will turn their intention into the desired behaviour (Adriaanse et al., 2011). Alternative behaviours to work on oneself naturally follow from learning about the vulnerability cycle with parents (Scheinkman & Dekoven Fishbane, 2004). Parents learn what behaviour of the other parent makes them have vulnerable, negative thoughts about themselves, and how they can strengthen themselves. This enables parents to choose a different behaviour than the automatic survival behaviour that they normally show in reaction to the other parent. In the group, this comes up frequently when parents interrogate each other about "plan B". Plan A is: "He will bring the children back in time; if not, I will start to panic and get furious". Plan B is: "I can count on him to bring the children back late, because that has always been the case. It is good for the children when I stop arguing about that, so I am going to enjoy watching a series until they arrive".

The joint start with parents and children can also help parents to be less sensitive and impulsive when reacting to the other parent. When PTSD has been diagnosed in a parent which is related to the ex-partner or to other life events, an extra trauma treatment may be an option, for instance EMDR (Eye Movement Desensitization and Reprocessing).

3.4.3 The importance of the social network

A unique element of the No Kids in the Middle treatment is the attention given to the social network. Research shows that, on average, parents in a conflict divorce are younger and have had shorter relationships than "normal" divorced parents. This could also mean that less trust has been built between parents and their social networks during the relationship. Paying explicit attention to building bridges of trust between both social networks may boost trust between parents.

Parents report that No Kids in the Middle does not change their perception of social network disapproval of the other parent. It does appear, though, that perceived social network disapproval is positively associated with the level of co-parenting conflicts. And this positive link is mediated by the tendency to forgive (see section 3.2.5). And although

No Kids in the Middle involves the social network in the treatment, the friends and relatives involved have not yet been interviewed and we do not know if the intervention has had an effect on them. Meanwhile, No Kids in the Middle has increasingly been targeting the social network. Parents are encouraged to do and share their homework with key people around them. We also invite members of the network more often in a crisis situation, if the parents are stuck, and in evaluations, too.

For the future, it is important to interview parents, children, the social network and providers about their perception of the different relationships in the system and about possible changes after No Kids in the Middle. HCD parents form a very complex group to work with and to study. Here, complexity and mutual influences on all levels of the system play an important role.

For children and adolescents, school is an important third social environment. Two-thirds of the older children suffer from the divorce when learning in school. Younger children especially receive a lot of support from confidential advisors at school – someone to whom they can confide their worries. But not all children have such an advisor. Chances for children to find such a source of support will be higher if the parents stimulate contacts between the child and school. The therapists can, for instance, advise the parents to inform school about the divorce. In addition, they can hear the child's voice even better by contacting school and the confidential adviser or by talking to a tutor. Naturally, this can only be done after the child (and parents) have agreed to such actions.

For older children, in particular, a good friend is their main source of support. It may be an option to arrange for a talk during the intervention between an adolescent who needs extra support and a friend. For adolescents without a source of support, the buddy project of Villa Pinedo (www.villapinedo.nl) may help strengthen their sense of belonging somewhere. This project pairs an experience expert of Villa Pinedo with a young person with divorced parents for support and recognition.

3.4.4 Parent-child and child-parent relationships

In the parent-child relationship we did not find any changes reported by parents and children. Parents reported that they had a good relationship with their children, they thought that they were available for their children and they had the impression that their children think they matter to their parents. In general, children also reported that they have a good relationship with their parents and that they can talk about their worries with them. We asked children to assess their mother and father separately.

The high scores in the pre measure may be the reason why parents and children did not experience any change. Children, however, do have stress-related complaints. Parents, in particular, attribute the stress to the other parent. It is very conceivable that children have a good relationship with each parent separately, but that tension and stress rise at the very moments when parents are together (see previous explanation). The transition between houses and the difference in rules in both houses is especially hard for children, and parents wrongly interpret their children's stress in these situations. Lagattuta, Sayfan and Bamford (2012), for instance, showed that parents underestimate the worries of these children and overestimate their optimism.

Parental reports about their children often show biases (López-Pérez & Wilson, 2015), and the biases of the fathers may be different from those of the mothers (De Los Reyes & Kazdin, 2005; Treutler & Epkins, 2003). It is therefore all the more important that children report themselves about their thoughts, behaviour and emotions, and that parents learn to take on the perspective of their children. The training provided by young people of Villa Pinedo to parents focuses exactly on taking on the perspective of the children (www.villapinedo.nl).

Follow-up research should not only be about pairing the parents' and children's experiences to further our understanding of how parents and children influence each other. It should also zoom in on how children perceive their parents when they are together, and also if children feel seen when they talk about the other house or the other parent or stepparent.

Compartmentalization

One-third of the children report that they feel they have to choose between their father and their mother. Literature shows that such compartmentalization – the shielding of one aspect of the self (here, the mother-child relationship) from another aspect of the self (here, the father-child relationship) – enables people to have a positive but unstable self-image. That self-image, however, is vulnerable to daily life stress and problems (Diehl & Hay, 2010; Showers & Zeigler-Hill, 2007). The integration of different aspects of the self and, in the case of divorced parents, an integrated representation of the family and the parents together, can make children less vulnerable to emotional and behavioural problems.

3.4.5 Changes in children of HCD parents

It is remarkable that children report a high level of well-being and a good relationship with their father and their mother, even though all families have been referred because the children's development and mental health are threatened by the interparental conflicts, and the results indicate that half of the children run an increased risk of developing PTSD. We have two possible explanations for these apparently conflicting results.

First, at the start of the intervention, the children mention that they have a difficult time, in particular, in the interspace. After the programme, we did ask the children if parents argue less, but not if the stress in the interspace had reduced. More research is needed into that.

Second, we asked the children to fill out the questionnaire in session 1 of the intervention. During this session, parents are also present in the parent group. We did this deliberately to avoid children filling out the questionnaire from the truth they live in when they are with one of the parents, that is, when only one of the parents is present. We hadn't considered, however, that the first meeting in itself may be very hopeful for the children. They see their parents together in the same room and they see that their parents are motivated to improve the situation for the children. Hope can make the children complete the forms more positively and optimistically.

Maybe parentification plays a role. Parentification means that a young person takes on the role of a parent for a long time with the corresponding tasks and responsibilities. Parentification is more prevalent in high-conflict divorce families (Hetherington & Elmore, 2003). The children may have learned to adjust to the situation with divorced parents and show resilient behaviour for the sake of the family. Maybe they failed to adequately learn to dwell on their own feelings. Their own feelings may be negatively biased, especially in relation to and when confronted by **both** parents (e.g. handovers and birthdays), and some measure of parentification may contribute to a premature development and resilience of children in divorce situations.

Strong parentified behaviour, however, often goes hand in hand with behavioural problems, low self-esteem and inferior social skills. It is only when children come of age that they grow more considerate towards themselves and take a new position towards the parents and the family (Van Parys et al., 2015). So, although children may now feel that they have a good life and a good relationship with their parents, it is possible that later on in their lives they will develop all kinds of problems related to too much responsibility and too much caring for the well-being of the parents in their childhood.

The number of children with a high risk of PTSD was just as high as the risk in a sample of physically abused children (Alisic et al., 2014). After following the No Kids in the Middle programme, less children had clinical scores, but the improvement was not significant. Part of the children showed an increased risk of PTSD in the pre measure and not in the post measure (20%); and part of the children did not have an increased risk in the pre measure, but they did in the post measure (7%). It is common knowledge that post-traumatic stress complaints sometimes intensify when the context becomes more peaceful (Andrews et al., 2007). Another explanation may be that the children's group was not a trauma-oriented treatment, but a group in which children were encouraged to share their thoughts and feelings regarding the divorce with each other. Developing a narrative (writing or acting out an own story about the event) to process traumatic events, however, is an important part of trauma treatment in children (Cohen et al., 2012). More research is needed to map out to what extent the children's groups of No Kids in the Middle can help children cope with traumatic experiences related to the divorce.

Other protective mechanisms may also be at play. Some of the existing literature suggests that children benefit from social role models in a stressful context (Chen & Miller, 2012). Such role models may help children accept stressors and to develop strategies which are required to get the best out of the situation and to adjust to the situation (so-called shifting strategies). Role models can also help children sustain optimism and hope, and not to give up when things work out badly (so-called persisting strategies). In our research, we could only demonstrate that children share their worries with others, but more research is needed to map out the protective functions of the social network of children.

Our findings suggest that children of divorced parents are not passive beings who just undergo parental conflicts. On the contrary, the children give their own meaning to what happens and we will only understand the interplay of parental conflicts in divorces and the well-being of children if the children, their opinion, feelings and thoughts are considered. In order to understand how children are affected by a divorce and the parental conflicts and disputes, it is important to examine what parents and the divorce mean to children. To date, however, little research has been done into this. With our research we have made a start.

As detailed in Chapters 6 and 9, we talk with the children about the interspace, both in the intake interview and in the group. We try to find out what exactly bothers the child and what goes well. Then, we support the child and, where possible, we talk with the parents about what they can do to reduce stress in the children. If parents continue to fight, we try to make the child more resilient in dealing with stress, and the children also give each other tips about dealing with stress.

We start the parent and the children's group together, as it helps to make the physical part of the interspace visible, tangible and, as such, a subject of discussion with parents and children. We start together with an exercise and then the children go to their own room. In the children's group, the therapists will ask: "Who of you could not decide who to sit next to, mum or dad?" "What do you do in that situation?" "How do you solve that problem?" The children get to talk about this and can give each other tips.

After conferring with the children, we talk about the answers from the children's group in the parent group. The following issues have become regular themes in the children group:

- How is the contact with both parents, how do parents deal with the interspace and how do children experience that?
- What goes well, what do parents do well and how can you tell?
- Who can the children talk to about what bothers them? Who in the family's social network supports them?
- Where do they suffer from the parental conflicts? At home, in school, with friends or somewhere else?
- When do they suffer less from the conflicts and why is that?
- How can they suffer less from the tensions?
- Can children give each other tips? For instance, suggesting breathing and physical exercises.

Like in the parent group, we focus on the positive experiences of the children. What goes well between parents, what do the children do differently themselves? We make sure that they enjoy being in the group and that they feel seen, heard and supported.

It is important to tell parents that research has shown that after following the No Kids in the Middle programme, parents have fewer conflicts and children feel that their parents argue less. This may encourage parents to participate in the therapy.

3.4.6 Research strengths and limitations

The study cautiously suggests a change in parents which may be related to participation in No Kids in the Middle: parents and children report a decrease in parental conflicts, parents indicate that the conflicts become more constructive, that they start to accept the divorce better and that they tend to forgive each other more. But change has not been shown in all intra and interpersonal domains of parents towards each other, nor have positive changes been reported in all domains of the children's functioning. Although children score high on well-being, it seems, in particular, that we have not sufficiently asked about what children suffer from in the divorce, in the so-called interspace.

To enhance our understanding of how parents, children and their network experience the No Kids in the Middle programme, and what does and what doesn't work, it is important to approach them as "fellow researchers". For instance, we can examine how effectiveness can be increased for as many families as possible by using feedback forms and in-depth interviews (Hennik & Hillewaere, 2017).

Questions we still have include: Which children run the highest risk of post-traumatic stress disorder? Why do children feel guilty about the divorce and the parental conflicts? Do children feel better if they are parentified? Does it help if children forgive their parents? Can children forgive their parents if parents forgive each other? How does the social network contribute to reducing parental conflicts? Can children start to feel better if they have someone who trusts them? How do the keystones of No Kids in the Middle (see Chapter 5) contribute to the better functioning of parents, children and their networks?

As mentioned before, the changes we have found in the current study may also be explained by other events taking place in the interspace. Furthermore, it is important to map out to what extent factors related to following the No Kids in the Middle programme, such as discontinuation of the legal proceedings, affect the current findings.

We have managed to reach a large and varied group of parents and children to participate in our study. We have included institutions who approached us with the request to participate. This, among other things, made employees of these institutions highly engaged in the research study. But, as always, we need to be cautious when drawing conclusions from the outcome of this study. It teaches us things and we use these learning experiences when we work with children, parents and the network, and also in cooperating with teams and further developing the programme. In the future, the voices of children and parents themselves and of their network, too, can play a bigger role in that.

Compared to other research studies, a remarkably high number of fathers have participated. This may have something to do with the personal and emotional subject of the study. Since so many fathers participated, we could compare the results of the fathers with those of the mothers. We see very few differences between men and women, which suggests that many processes work the same for both.

Part 2

Practice

Chapter 4

Methodology outline

The programme is intended for parents who do not live together and cannot reach consensus on a good parenting plan (Cottyn, 2009) and continue to fight about issues like care for the children, living and money.

GOAL

The goal of the treatment is to help the parents reduce the tensions between them so that they can provide a safe parenting climate that is "good enough" for their children – a climate in which parents have enough trust to focus on optimizing their own situation and where they can better accept differences with the other parent so that the tensions between the them will reduce. It is about de-escalating the battle and making sure that the children are central again.

The methodology is described so that the framework and keystones of the intervention are clear, but also so that there is room to tailor to specific needs. That means that adjustments can be made which fit the needs of the clients we work with and also those of the therapists conducting the programme. We therefore like to emphasize that the methodology of No Kids in the Middle is a "living framework" – a process to inspire colleagues to work in a similar way. It is not a recipe book prescribing exactly what should be done in which session for how many minutes. It is more like a cook giving instructions: "Just taste now and then decide whether you need another handful of spices or a splash of cream". The composition of the program has proven to be effective. The themes link up well with each other and help parents to de-escalate and to really see their children again.

The programme starts by building a proper working relationship and increasing the sense of safety. This helps parents and children build confidence in the treatment, in one another and themselves. This allows them to reflect on new possibilities. The participants first get to know each other and share information and make contact before touching on stress-inducing themes.

In doing so, we use a number of theoretical assumptions which can help stop the battle and create a safer environment for all of the people involved. We see theoretical assumptions as auxiliary frameworks, not as descriptions of the truth.

A theory which helps to move from a destructive to a more constructive interaction is a good starting point. Bateson (1972) tackles this theme in *Steps to an Ecology of Mind*, in which he explains that the territory never exactly corresponds with the map of that area ("the map is not the territory"). He also explains that the value of a map is not determined by the reliability of the reproduction of that area (the reality) but rather by its usability, since the structure of the map is useful for the particular goal. In terms of our programme, we have looked for a usable theory for our goal: de-escalating the battle between the parents and promoting a safe environment in which parents can relax and children can grow up.

The theory of the methodology is covered in the first three group sessions. The first session deals with destructive patterns and spirals of fight (session 1), the second with the effects of fighting parents on children (session 2), and the third session is about the destructive power of demonizing stories and how to bend them into more connecting stories with which children can live (session 3). Throughout all the sessions, there is attention to de-escalation, vulnerabilities, trauma reactions and the window of tolerance. In Chapter 8, which describes the sessions, we explain how the theory is embedded in the therapy and how it can be used in the group.

In the children's group we work with themes. We listen to the children and support them in composing a coherent story about their lives and the divorce. In this way, they can better deal with the stress of parents in conflict. If the parents manage to reduce or stop the battle and to create a peaceful and safe environment for their child again, this life story may also help in dealing with trauma. If children are not ready to talk, play, draw or express themselves about the conflicts and the divorce, this is not needed.

4.1 Main characteristics of the treatment

Six families are treated at the same time. We work in two groups, a parent group and a children's group. Each session starts with a warm-up for the children, parents and therapists together.

Before the treatment starts, parents and children go through an intake process. The first exploratory talk is with the parents only. We prefer parents come together. If parents are triggered so much by the other that too much stress makes it impossible for them to digest information and to weigh things when they are together, it is possible to come separately. After this first talk, parents always come together.

If after the exploratory talk parents decide to enrol, an intake interview will be scheduled for the children and parents together. This intake interview serves to get acquainted with the children, to learn something about their lives and to explain to them what the children's group is about. With the parents, we will talk about their wounds and where they get stuck.

After the intake process, the parent group and the children's group come together eight times for two hours at the same point in time, once every two weeks. There are two therapists for the parent group and two for the children's group. We also strive to have one trainee in each group. This means that for each group of families, six therapists work together. The therapists support and help each other, too.

The children (in principle, all the children of the parents joining the programme) follow their own programme. In the children's group, themes are tackled that are relevant for all children of divorced parents. Apart from talking about these themes, the children work on a creative presentation for the parents in which they show what they experience as a child of parents in conflict. The presentations can be about the troubles or the worries of the children, but also about what goes well and about their wishes.

In the parent group we explain the demonizing patterns in their communication, how the stress system works, dealing with emotions within the window of tolerance, the direct and indirect consequences for children, and the destructive power of dominant and demonizing stories. We provide this information together and in dialogue with the parents. We avoid a "pedagogical" tone. In the dialogue, parents do not only learn from the therapists, but also from each other, and the therapists also learn from the parents. It strengthens the parents in their position as a parent when they figure out together what the children in their situation need and how they can provide for those needs as parents.

In addition to providing information and reflecting, we do a lot of exercises related to important themes. When parents get stuck, we look for new possibilities.

In session six, the children present the results of their creative group work to the parents and therapists. In the same session or in session seven, parents present what they have learned from the programme and what they wish for their children in the future to the children and therapists.

After the group session, the therapists will have a subsequent discussion.

4.2 Session outline

The following table provides a more detailed outline of the stages involved in the sessions.

	Parents	*Children*	*Story about the family and the divorce*
Preliminary	Both parents enrol (see Appendix 1). Invitation by No Kids in the Middle for an exploratory talk	–	
Exploratory talk	Getting acquainted Explanation of programme • conditions • willingness to work to change oneself • importance of the network meeting • no legal proceedings Questions of parents Agreement on participation or not If so: • complete registration form • complete form with open questions (see Appendix 2) • mail referral letter in child's name • copy of child's identity card • approval to request information from previous social workers • informed consent to participate in scientific research (optional)	Not present	

Intake	Therapists and family get acquainted Participation of the children Discuss with parents: • what do parents want to change in themselves? • impeding factors • who will come to the network meeting? In parallel, an individual talk with both parents and one of the parent therapists about wounds in the past and triggers in the present Therapists discuss with each other what they have understood from the parents while the parents listen Parents receive/buy *A Workbook for the "No Kids in the Middle" Intervention Programme* Get moving: see Homework for session 1, *A Workbook for the "No Kids in the Middle" Intervention Programme* Clinical questionnaires about problems in children and parents are filled out before the start of session 1	Getting acquainted Explanation of the children's group The two houses and the interspace Give children a voice and look for strengths Optional: Clinical questionnaires	Drawing or photo of the two houses and the interspace
Network meeting	Explanation of programme and methodology Presentation by young experience experts of Villa Pinedo Questions from the network Calling in help from the network	Not present	

(*Continued*)

(Continued)

	Parents	*Children*	*Story about the family and the divorce*
Session 1	Welcome Joint warm-up with parents and children Positive memories Explanation of destructive communication patterns Exercise on destructive patterns Get moving: see Homework for session 2, *A Workbook for the "No Kids in the Middle" Intervention Programme* Closing words	Warm-up Getting acquainted Theme: the two houses and the interspace Making a creative presentation for the parents or working on their perception of what goes well and what they feel when their parents are fighting	A brief outline of the current situation of each child Who live(s) in which house and since when? When is the child where and with whom? The story of the family and the divorce is only composed if children want it and feel safe enough This may vary per session. Match the child's pace!
Session 2	Warm-up What has changed since last time (especially to the better)? Exercise on child's role, in three different rounds Review of the three home assignments: what did the parents do and how did the network respond? Discuss consequences for children Get moving: see Homework for session 3, *A Workbook for the "No Kids in the Middle" Intervention Programme* Closing words	Warm-up Theme: one house with both parents – how did it start between the parents and what was nice? Continue working on the presentation	A brief outline of the start of each child's life How did parents get to know each other and when were the children born? What was nice in the beginning?
Session 3	Warm-up Story for the children about the divorce Explanation (or reading at home) of traumas, conflicts and the stress system Group discussion and reflection Get moving: see Homework for session 4, *A Workbook for the "No Kids in the Middle" Intervention Programme* Closing words	Warm-up Theme: tensions between parents, loyalty and choosing Continue working on the presentation	A brief outline of what goes right and wrong between the parents of each child. Why did the parents get a divorce? What do the children find difficult?

Session 4	Warm-up What has changed for the better? Review homework, round of symbols and compliments Issues: new solutions to old problems Get moving: see Homework for session 5, *A Workbook for the "No Kids in the Middle" Intervention Programme* Closing words	Warm-up Have the children noticed any changes at home? Theme: tensions between parents, reactions of children What do you do if parents have conflicts? Do children wish to share something about the worst thing they have experienced? Continue working on the presentation	A brief outline of the disputes or tensions which each child still has to think about. How can the child cope with these tensions?
Session 5	Warm-up How did parents do the assignments they gave themselves? What has changed for the better at home? Issues: moving again after stagnated conflicts Get moving: see Homework for session 6 *A Workbook for the "No Kids in the Middle" Intervention Programme* Closing words	Warm-up Theme: resilience and unfinished themes from previous sessions Continue working on the presentation	Skills and strengths of each child
Session 6	Preparing the presentations for the children Presentations from children to parents Reflections and feelings when watching the presentations Continue working on issues Get moving: see Homework for session 7, *A Workbook for the "No Kids in the Middle" Intervention Programme* Closing words	Preparing presentations Presentations to parents Talking about how they felt during the presentations and zooming in on reactions of parents in a positive way Game	

(*Continued*)

(Continued)

	Parents	*Children*	*Story about the family and the divorce*
Session 7	Preparing parent presentations and receiving the children Presentations of the parents to the children Talking about how it felt to give the presentation Continue working on issues Get moving: see Homework for session 8, *A Workbook for the "No Kids in the Middle" Intervention Programme* Closing words	Have children noticed any changes at home? Parent presentations Talking about the presentations and zooming in on the positive intentions of parents for the children Game	
Session 8	Warm-up Evaluation and closure	Warm-up Theme: tips and goodbye	Taking the story about the divorce home (optional)
Evaluation	Talk with both parents, the children and key people from the network		

4.3 Safety and change

In recent years, the news has told the story of a number of families with parents who had been involved in a divorce battle for years and the situation ended with one parent killing the children and him/herself. These shocking events arouse indignation, distress, anger and concerns, and it raises the question if such family tragedies can be avoided. Often, risk assessments are considered: assessing the risk that someone will (again) exhibit violent behaviour in the future. Assessing the risk that a family tragedy will occur is extremely difficult.Verheugt (2007) conducted research into child murders by parents and came to the conclusion that they often come as a surprise. There need not have been a history of violence or psychopathy. What he did find were a lot of parental traumatic childhood experiences, often related to the absence of the parents and experiences of loss. A divorce can re-open these old wounds.

Preventing family tragedies is therefore more a matter of recognizing old wounds in parents than being aware of criminal or violent behaviour. In the programme, we see a lot of wounds, traumas and loss in parents, but rather than performing a risk assessment, we want to gain insight into the possibility that parents will de-escalate and change to create a safer environment for the children, for each other and for themselves. Or, as Harnett calls it, the "capacity to change" (Harnett, 2007). He proposes a framework to work on the development of a safe parenting climate for children and which enables us to assess if parents are capable and willing enough to change and benefit from the treatment. Asen (2016) calls it "therapeutic assessment". For this therapeutic assessment, the children's voice is leading for us. They may say and show us that the atmosphere at home has become more relaxed and that they feel seen and heard.

A risk assessment may illuminate risk factors. Still, although a lot of social workers had been involved with these families, too, and dangers had been assessed, things went wrong all the same. Dijkstra and Verhoeven (2014) investigated a family tragedy and they arrived, among other things, at the following recommendations:

- Effort should be put into these families to ease the fierce battle, with attention towards the strong emotions.
- Violence must be concretized and specified.
- Efforts should be put into increasing safety and the well-being of the children must be systematically strengthened.

These three points are addressed in No Kids in the Middle. This becomes clear from the description of the intake interview and the sessions. From the very first contact, we point out to parents that they are responsible for the children. The children are caught in the battle and the parents are going to join No Kids in the Middle to change this. For that purpose, they need to change their behaviour as parents, and that is what we follow as therapists.

We deliberately choose to not perform a risk assessment. Specifically in high-conflict divorces, stress levels are very high in both parents and each attempt to measure the safety with instruments may increase this stress in the parents, the children and the professionals. Another thing is that the outcomes are snapshots in time, which are biased by the escalating divorce battle. Completing risk assessment forms suggests carefulness, while it doesn't help to increase safety.

Hurst (2011) also points out the dangers of too much confidence in risk assessments. They formalize the contact with clients and there is no conclusive evidence that the instruments really predict risk (Hurst, 2011). He also pleads for the return of the clinical assessment made in contacts with clients, and for acceptance of a certain degree of uncertainty. If we cannot accept doubt, Hurst says, fear will paralyze our practices. It is precisely this fear that makes us less effective. He describes how safety in a family can be assessed in a systematic and narrative way through dialogue with the family members.

Thanks to years of clinical experience, the professional often recognizes signs of risk. It is important to take these signs seriously. One part of the No Kids in the Middle methodology revolves around discussing risk signs and concerns about the safety in face-to-face contact with the parents. If children above 12 years of age are involved, this is, of course, also discussed with the children themselves. The responsibility for safety is placed on the parents and is not without obligations. We ask the parents if they recognize the concerns and what they are going to do to take the concerns away. In the next session, we talk about what parents have actually done and if this has taken away the concerns. The treatment team considers which of the therapists will talk about the concerns with parents and children. We aim for optimal transparency and do not "save up" concerns before talking about them.

An example is a boy who constantly makes remarks and gestures with a sexual overtone in the first session of the children's group. This causes unease in the group and raises concerns among the child therapists. Immediately, in that same week, one of the child therapists and one of the parent therapists talk about this behaviour and the concerns it raises with the parents. We ask if they recognize the behaviour and if they share our concerns. They are surprised and glad that we addressed this issue face to face with them. They are open to investigating the reason for this behaviour. It turns out that, because of a lack of space, the adolescent sleeps in his mother's room, together with his sisters. This excites him too much. The mother decides to change this and to talk about it with her son. The father promises to talk with his son about his sexual development and to support him in that. The annoying and worrisome behaviour did not recur in the group after that. In this example, the parents could reassure the therapists. This, too, is a clinical assessment where the inner dialogue of the therapist is paramount. If concerns continue to exist, the therapist team will consider possible follow-up steps.

The five steps of the basic model for development of a reporting code for domestic violence and child abuse are leading:

1 Mapping out signs.
2 Consulting with a colleague and, optionally, a child protection service.
3 Talking with the clients.
4 Assessing domestic violence or child abuse:
   (a) Based on steps 1 through 3, do I suspect domestic violence or child abuse?
   (b) Do I suspect acute or structural unsafety?
5 Make two decisions:
   (a) Is it necessary to report the case to a child protection service?
   (b) Is it also possible to offer or arrange for (adequate) help yourself?

In case of current accusations of violence or current signs, multiple disciplines will work together to sort out the situation as best they can and to restore safety.

We have to be continuously aware that we cannot check the truth. Unfortunately, we cannot guarantee safety for children. What we can do, however, is use our professional expertise, experience and clinical intuition, make it explicit and share it with colleagues, parents and children. We can cooperate with parents and their networks to enhance the safety for children as much as possible.

4.4 Therapists

What does this require from the therapists?

Education/training

- To be able to conduct this therapeutic groupwork, therapists must have received preparatory training in systemic therapy and been trained in recognizing and treating trauma and stress reactions in children and adults. Then, they must participate in the three-day training of No Kids in the Middle and, together with their team, conduct their first group programme, which will be supervised.

Attitude

- The programme requires therapists who like to work together in a team and enjoy working on these problems with families in groups.
- It requires the personal strength and presence of the therapists. They must be able to deal with intense conflicts and emotional reactions without going under themselves.
- Therapists of No Kids in the Middle care a lot about children and like to work with them. At the same time, they are not condemning towards parents. They actively look for the good in the parent and also recognize the "wounded child" in the parent. They can take the side of the parents to help the children and do not walk into the trap of being the "better parent" themselves. They can protect children and, at the same time, recognize and strengthen their resilience.

Teams

- Teams working together with this target group must maintain their attention on safety. Therapists may feel vulnerable or become moved when working with these families. Then, a safe cooperative team is the best context to stay strong. Therapists do not need to be able to do all this from the start. It is precisely in a safe team where people usually learn a lot and learn fast. Room for intervision is essential here, though.

Exchange of knowledge and experience

- To stay motivated and abreast of developments, a "working community" of therapists working with the group programme who are committed and continue to participate in intervision, attend follow-up days and refresher courses is needed. New developments and ideas can be shared in the working community which can serve as fuel for further development of the No Kids in the Middle methodology.

Support by the management

- The organization that incorporates No Kids in the Middle as a form of treatment in their treatment package must support this group treatment and the therapists working with it. They must also provide time for intervision and consultation. Managers are advised to attend a training session of No Kids in the Middle once.

4.5 The groups, general organization

4.5.1 Preliminary and subsequent discussions and break

Preparing rooms

The therapists of the parent and children's group meet at least half an hour before the group session. During this half hour, the rooms are prepared for the work. In the parent group, 14 chairs are placed in a circle, preferably leaving an open space in the middle. There is always a flip-chart or a whiteboard available in the room. There are also sheets of paper and felt-tip pens for exercises, if any. At some distance, there is a desk and a chair for the student writing the reports and operating the video camera.

In the room where the children's group gathers, there are mats and/or cushions on the floor and there may also be some chairs. In addition, there is material to work with, such as paper and felt-tip pens, paint, coloured chalks, a video/photo camera, dress-up clothes and other things to play with. There is also a corner where children can chill out and watch, for instance, a film. This often proves to be necessary, because a two-hour session is quite long for the younger children, especially since the sessions take place after school. There is also a seat for a student to operate the camera and to make notes. In the children's group, the student also frequently works with the children him/herself.

If possible, the rooms for the children's and the parent group are close to each other. We have noticed that it works well for parents if the children can be heard now and then, like their footsteps or laughter. Obviously, the children should not be able to hear what is said in the parent group. Preferably, a separate waiting and break room is available for the six families: the family room. The therapists prepare this room and make sure that there is something to drink (tea, coffee, water, lemonade) and that there is fruit available. Preferably no cookies or candy, as it often makes children very active.

Preliminary discussion

After all these preparations, there are usually ten to 15 minutes left to get together and briefly go through the schedule or share important information about, for instance, a parent or a child not being able to attend, a school that has called out of concern, a parent who has sent a concerned or angry email, and so on.

Arrival

After arrival, parents and children go to the family room. If there is no separate family room, they wait together in the waiting room. Usually, one of the parents arrives with the children and the other parent arrives alone. The parents arriving with the children usually feel more protected. The parents arriving alone feel less safe. Tension is often electric in the waiting room, but the mix of six families makes the tension bearable. The therapists of the parent group and of the children's group invite the parents and children to the room where the warming up takes place.

Break

Halfway through the session, both groups have a break. Both the parents and the children need a break. And it is time in which parents and children can be together without therapists or a programme. The therapists need the break to coordinate things between the groups. The pace in the parent group determines the exact moment of the break. One of the parent therapists will go to the children's group to announce the break. In this way, children never have to wait for the parents in the break room and they cannot listen to and hear what is said in the parent room.

Especially in the beginning, children appear to be very concerned about what happens in the parent room. When a therapist came to announce the break, seven-year-old Kevin immediately asked the therapist if his parents had already been arguing downstairs. "Not at all", the therapist replied truthfully. "Well, you just wait and see", Kevin responded.

We ask the parents to watch over their children and to make sure that other people in the building will not be disturbed during the break. Parents and children stay in the family room or, if there is no such room, in a waiting room. The parents and children are there without therapists. A lot will happen in this room.

Children who haven't seen a parent for a long time will now see the parent. And many children will see their parents together in one room again, something they have not witnessed for a long time. Since the six families are there together, there is enough motion and space to ensure that the atmosphere does not become too tense. Sometimes children stay in the corridor or in a corner to avoid a parent, or parents go through a lot of trouble avoiding the other parent. But after a number of sessions, there will usually be a more relaxed atmosphere and less avoidance behaviour.

Parents also see how other parents get along with their children. Sometimes, they can appreciate the other parent again when they see how nice the other parent can be with other people. Or a mother sees how her little daughter crawls on her father's lap, where she assumed that her daughter was afraid of her dad. Things will change during the break and the therapists don't witness it, but it will become evident during the sessions.

The therapists sit together for 15 minutes and can briefly share how things are progressing and how they experience the process in their group.

Subsequent discussion

After each session, the therapists first tidy up the children's room, the parent room and the family room. Then, they look back on the session. In these 30 to 60 minutes they share their experiences, frustrations, grief and joy about the developments in the groups. The children's group is discussed first. Often, the therapists also briefly talk about the parents. Then, tasks will be divided, such as: asking parents for approval to get in touch with school, sending an email to a parent, talking to grandparents, and so on. Sometimes, an extra session is scheduled.

Important incidents are briefly mentioned. Often, some action needs to be taken after a session. A GP, guardian, school or child may need to be called or an email may need to be written. And there is always attention towards the parallel process between the parent group, the children's group and the team of therapists (see section 9.3.1). During the review, the student makes a to-do list for the next two weeks. All therapists will receive this list by email and the preliminary discussions are used to go over this list again. If there are worrying signs, an extra appointment may be scheduled with the therapists involved.

4.5.2 The warm-up

Each session starts with a warm-up, preferably in the room where the parents work. This makes for a light-hearted, relaxing start for the parents, children and therapists. The warm-ups are tailored to the theme in the children's group. Chapter 9, which is about the children's group, describes the various warm-up exercises.

4.5.3 Final report

We write a final report for each family taking part in the programme. The final report describes the main parts of the parent and children's group (see Appendix 5). Some parents want us to rewrite the final report because they do not recognize themselves or the other parent enough in it. Usually, these are the parents who, by the end of the treatment, still want the other parent to change. We always talk about the part dealing with the children in general terms with the children themselves, and we ask them if they agree with what we have written about them. We let the parents read the entire report. If the parents do not agree with the report, we invite them to add their reflections in the form of an appendix. See Appendices 6 and 7 for two example reports.

4.6 No Kids in the Middle as a first course, main course or dessert

Some of the families that come to see us have already received a lot of care. This care may be provided for just one or a few children, as is the case when they are placed in custody. In other families, there has been therapy in the form of, for instance, relational therapy for the parents, parent counselling, a post-divorce parenting course, trauma therapy for one or both parents or for the children, mediation or forensic mediation, and sometimes a combination of multiple interventions.

Dessert

The No Kids in the Middle programme may serve as a dessert that can build on all previous interventions. Sometimes, everything falls into place and parents can take a different path. They often start by saying: "This is our last straw. We have done so much already". Parents, their networks and especially the children may need a life with fewer fights so badly. They can be so fed up with the life energy and money that the battle has cost in all these years. Like a father said, with great emotion, after he had radically changed his behaviour in a session:

> It is only now that I realise how much life energy these eight years of battle have cost me. It has made me ill, I have lost a lot of money, I have lost a lot of friends. It has dominated my life, and why really?

It didn't help anyone. On the contrary! It is terrible to realise only now, but it also helps me to start living again.

Main course

Sometimes, the programme is a main course. In that case, there has been little help or care before, or each type of therapy has been stopped or has been used as part of the battle. Then, No Kids in the Middle can help parents and their networks to take a different path, getting kids out of the middle.

First course

For another group of families, No Kids in the Middle is a first course. These families take steps during the programme, but at the end of the eight sessions they have not found a new form where the kids are no longer in the middle. We offer these families follow-up care tailored to their needs. Preferably, the therapists of this group are tasked with the follow-up.

Some parents want further therapy, sometimes including a new partner or with another family member attending. Some parents are willing to consider trauma therapy or another individual therapy after No Kids in the Middle. Some families have additional meetings with the network. The therapists take responsibility by thinking along with the parents and, if needed, also finding good follow-up care. Preferably, the therapists engage in the (brief) follow-up themselves, which allows them to build on what has already been achieved. A parent therapist may continue to have talks with the parents, often with network members attending, too. Sometimes, a child or one of the parents needs some form of individual therapy after the programme. Sometimes, family talks with parents and children are a good continuation of the programme.

If a family is supervised and/or if other care is being provided, it is important to have contact with the relevant social and youth protection workers. We try to secure the increased activity and responsibility of the parents by adequately involving social workers and youth protection workers, and by informing them about what parents have learned.

We express our confidence in the potential of the parents themselves. If therapists still worry about a certain situation, they will mention this during the evaluation and discuss with the parents what is needed.

Some parents have put their legal proceedings on hold and have to go back to the lawyers to agree, for instance, on the covenant and the parenting plan or parental access. We hope that the lawyers will pick up the positive tone and support them. Sometimes, a telephone call helps to steer the lawyers in that direction.

Since we can provide this type of follow-up ourselves, we can build on what has already been covered and achieved in the group. Continuity of care is of utmost importance.

Chapter 5

The keystones

The No Kids in the Middle programme has a number of keystones. These keystone elements are typical of the programme and incorporate theoretic assumptions, clinical experiences and scientific findings. The elements are clearly very prominent in the implementation of the programme and support the programme.

The keystones relate to our hypotheses about what factors are effective in this programme. Whether they are indeed directly connected with these effective factors is a question for future research. For now, the initial findings of the scientific research (T1 and T2) and the follow-up measurement (T3) provide support for these hypotheses.

It is not easy to choose the right term for these keystones. We could call it basic elements, main characteristics, basic assumptions, foundations, keystones or fundamentals. We opt for the term keystones. It means, among other things, "a central cohesive source of support and stability". This clarifies exactly what we mean by these basic elements.

Figure 5.1 represents the keystones as interconnected cogs which are continuously moving and influencing each other. In that sense, there is no hierarchy. The keystones may alternately come to the forefront or stay in the background. This may depend on the context, cultural aspects, the team, the group or the issues between parents.

The keystones are basic foundations for the children, the parents, the network as well as the therapists. These are interrelated systems.

Three of the six keystones are about conditions:

1 *attitude*: the attitude adopted throughout the programme;
2 *community*: working in and with groups and communities; and
3 *children*: attention on the children and the *interspace*.

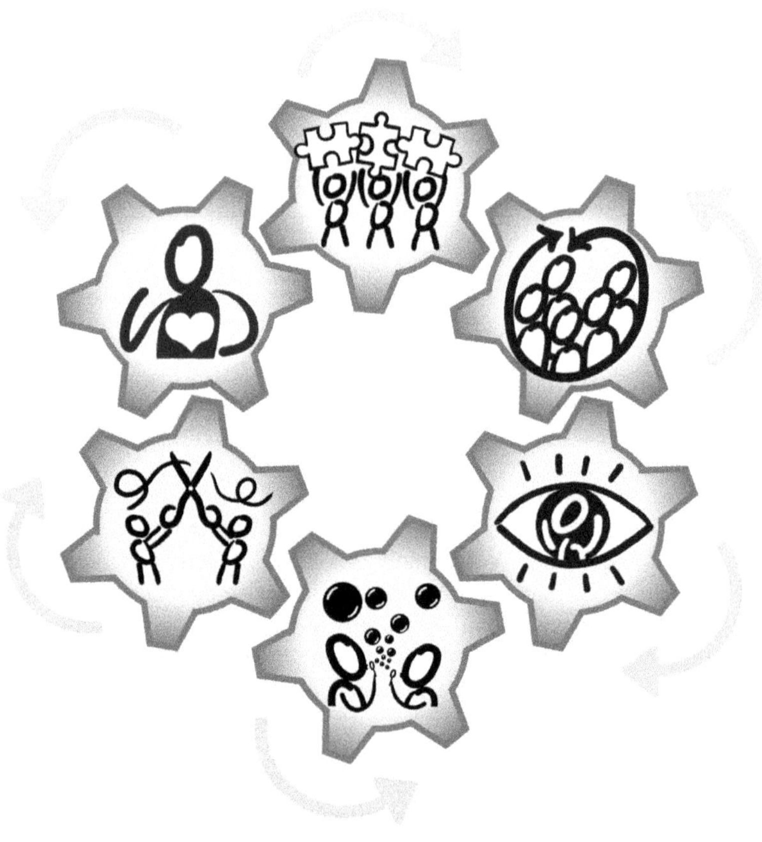

Figure 5.1 Keystones

The other three keystones concern the process of the treatment. They relate to the main parts of the intervention:

1 *Letting go*: letting go and making the transition to real separation and accepting differences. This relates to being able to accept tragedy, dealing with grief, being able to tolerate ambivalence and letting go of the illusion of control.
2 *Destructive patterns*: acknowledging and reducing destructive patterns and conflict spirals by recognizing them and connecting them with the vulnerability cycle (wounds, stress reactions, trauma and survival strategies). Working on emotion regulation.

3 *Changing by experiencing*: learning by action and performance (experiencing, feeling, acting, telling new stories, presenting).

The keystones form the framework and the basic structure of No Kids in the Middle. This structure allows room for variations and cultural adaptations. Therapists have room to work responsively, interacting with the parents, the children, the network and the team of therapists. They are driven by feedback. That means that the feedback of the people involved also determines the course of the therapeutic process.

No Kids in the Middle is not a fixed script, not a strict protocol. It is a live process that continuously takes on a different form. This allows the keystones to stand firm and provide stability.

5.1 Attitude

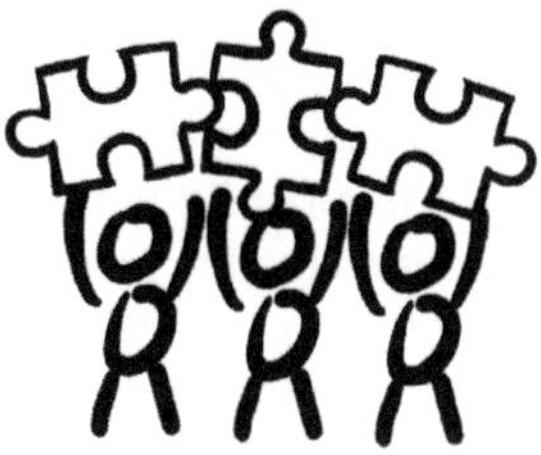

Working together

From the very start, the therapists try to build an atmosphere in which the entire group, parents and therapists alike work together to create a better situation for children, for themselves and the people around them. The therapists are there to connect. The parent therapists know the children by name and they frequently say something about the children. For instance, "It was nice to see that Sofie was snuggling up against you during the warm-up", or "How nice of Said to bring his guitar". The child therapists regularly say something to the children about their parents. For instance, "Dad was very proud of you when you showed him that drawing during the break", or "That was nice, sitting on your mother's lap, wasn't it?"

Ethical

Therapists take an ethical stand. That means that they aim for all those involved to be heard and to be done justice to. Any inequality and abuse of power, oppression of children, adults, parents or professionals is discouraged.

Non-judgemental, emphatic

Therapists do not judge parents, children or their network. Neither do they condemn each other. They make sure that they do not take the position of "the better parent" who does see the child, understands and protects them. The parents are recognized and supported in their position as a parent.

The therapists position themselves as professionals who do this work out of commitment to children and parents, with the aim of creating a safe environment so that everyone can progress. They start with the idea that there are ways forward in all families. They continue to express this confidence. They do not know how things will turn out for this family, but they will devote themselves to them. Therapists take the position of "safe uncertainty" (Mason, 1993). They radiate the confidence that they know what they are doing without knowing exactly how things will turn out for this family in the course of the treatment. In a safe way, they are insecure, creating an openness about the path the parents are going to take.

Parents who have been fighting for a long time have often barricaded themselves in their own positions and certainties. Both have a monopoly on their own conviction. They try to convince each other and their network of their own conviction. They are themselves in a state of "unsafe certainty" (Mason, 1993). If relatives or other people from the network challenge these parents or enter battle with them, this usually adds fuel to the flames.

The therapists always try to avoid this battle position. The starting point is a multi-partiality approach with the focus on the children. Sometimes this is difficult, so the therapists need each other to maintain this multi-partiality approach to make all voices heard and not to walk into the trap of condemnation or control. External control does not work for these desperate and suspicious parents.

Focus on possibilities

Parents often feel that they have already tried everything to solve the problems and that they are running out of options. To each suggestion, they say: "Yes, but" (I already tried that so many times, it's no good because . . . etc.). The therapists invite the parents to look for new possibilities together and to opt for

> YES, (for instance: we understand how painful it must be for you and that you have lost courage) AND (for instance: It can't go on like this for the children, can it, for you or the children. Shall we try to find a way for you to do things differently to improve the situation?).

The feeling of powerlessness is often connected with years of efforts to change the other person and to draw all those involved, including the social workers, into the situation. Since this is a dead-end street, these parents often feel dispirited and powerless. That feeling of powerlessness can often be broken by concentrating on their own behaviour. They will then see that change can open new possibilities.

When therapists are not sure how to continue or when they feel desperate themselves, they ask the group for help. For instance,

> We have a feeling that we have done something wrong, because the atmosphere in the group has become increasingly unsafe and we feel a great deal of pain and desperation. We are not sure how to move on without increasing the pain. Can you help us? Does anyone have a suggestion?

If this question is genuine, the group will always offer to help, which will stimulate a process towards a safer environment.

This position of the therapist as a relief seeker, as someone who is taking a closer look at himself and wants to change, is at odds with the dynamics of a high-conflict divorce and challenges the parents to stretch beyond the bounds of the impossible and to explore the landscape of possibilities together (Wilson, 2007).

When colleagues in the team feel powerless, they will look for possibilities together: a different perspective of the mother, another intervention, or just do nothing and wait.

We also look at possibilities with the children. For instance, what can they do to suffer less from the battle?

Structuring

Parents usually feel the need to tell what happened, to prove their point, to share the pain and to receive recognition for that. The therapists limit this by stopping the parent who wants to tell a lot of stories and give examples of misbehaviour by the other parent. The therapist acknowledges and stresses that it is only natural that everyone wants to share their story, but that there is no room for all the stories. This may increase stress levels in the group too much and inhibit a workable climate. The therapist will ask the parent to give one small example to clarify the story, using the metaphor that for a full-blood picture, no more than one drop of blood is needed.

The structure of the programme offers safety for clients and therapists, which allows the possibility to experiment with new behaviour. A safe structure is ensured and limits are set, both in the parent and in the children's group.

The team of therapists also needs structure: the structure of preliminary, interim and subsequent discussions, in which frustrations and vulnerabilities can also be expressed.

Present

A non-violent attitude and an attitude of being present (Omer, 2007), where using emotional or physical violence is not accepted and exceeding relational limits is discouraged, is just as important as empathizing and acknowledging pain. Presence and empathy are inseparable. Just like supporting children, protecting them where possible and building resilience are inseparable.

The therapists do not pressure the children or the parents to discuss certain issues or to answer questions. There is room for silence, hesitation and doubt. The attitude of the therapists is inviting, but not commanding. Therapists do not ask the parents to become a cooperative team, as this may aggravate the conflicts. The therapists are open to parallel parenting where parents let go of each other and leave each other alone as much as possible.

Responsibility

The therapists do not check on or punish the parents, but they do remind them of their responsibilities. They ask the parents to write down for themselves what they want to achieve and what they wish for their children, themselves and the people who love them. If parents try to put the blame for the misery on anyone but themselves, the therapists will challenge them to look at what they can do themselves to change the situation. The parents will get homework assignments, which they are supposed to do with the people around them. In the group, we discuss what they have done with the assignments and what can be yielded from it.

Therapists, too, take responsibility. For instance, by being there on time, being committed and present, by answering emails and supporting colleagues. Therapists are also prepared to take a close look at their own behaviour or vulnerabilities and what they do to them. They support each other in that.

Therapists make room for hope for change, but hope must match the possibilities. When the hope for positive change does not match the possibilities, this will pave the way for disappointment in children, parents, the network and themselves. Disappointment can again lead to escalation of the demonizing processes. The therapists make clear that success is not guaranteed and that the desired change may not be achieved.

5.2 Community

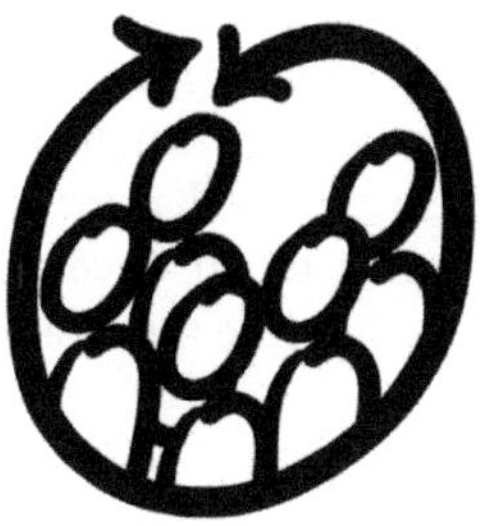

Working in and with groups

In the No Kids in the Middle programme, we have chosen to work in groups because change processes often stagnate when working with individual families (divorced parents and their children). Groups and communities form a context for multiple voices and dialogue. In a group, parents learn from each other; they support each other like the children in the children's group also support and encourage each other.

Children benefit from peer support. They become more in touch with their perception, their feelings and their story, which makes them stronger and boosts their resilience. Even though they do not necessarily have to express themselves, they are able to better understand what is going on and how they feel. The fact that the parent and the children's group sessions run parallel allows children to see that parents are working. This releases them from guilt and it will relieve their mind.

Parents are a mirror to each other, find acknowledgment and recognition in the group, and can support each other in finding an alternative route. They have a network around them with a new partner, grandparents, relatives and friends. They also have professionals such as teachers, the GP, lawyers, social workers, mediators and others. These networks can intensify conflicts and make them escalate, but they can also ease them and make them de-escalate. We actively look for ways of cooperation with the personal and professional network to reduce conflicts.

The therapists work in a team. They learn from each other and support each other. If one of them feels powerless, another one will still see possibilities. Or if a therapist gets annoyed with a parent, the other therapist will still be able to empathize with that parent. Both the child and the parent therapist may be greatly moved during the treatment process. In the therapist team there is room to deal with this. This ensures and strengthens the resilience of the therapists, while it requires a relationship based on mutual trust. Therapists must be able to trust each other and feel confirmation that the other appreciates and recognizes them in their professionalism. It goes hand in hand with a feeling of solidarity and sympathy, and requires a good relationship between the therapists working together since these groups demand a lot from the therapist.

Therapeutic presence also means that the therapists work as a team and keep each other informed of all developments. In the children's group, things may come up which the therapists of the parent group need to know, and vice versa.

This needs to be done with great care. We make sure that the comments made by the children do not become ammunition in the battle and are not used against them. If children, for instance, mention that the previous weekend at their mother's was not a pleasant one because their mother had been arguing with their stepfather, then it is good to know about that, but it is not good to directly tackle the mother about it. On the other hand, such information may be thematized in the children's group:

> "Does your mother/father ever argue with your stepparent? How do you cope with that? Can you talk about it? With whom?"

And also in the parent group:

> "Is there any arguing in the families? Can children just say that they don't like it? How do other parents deal with that?"

In the battle dynamics, forces often play a part which may drive a wedge between the team members. This should be avoided at all times. For the coherence of the team it is very important that therapists keep each other informed and, where possible, make tensions a subject of discussion.

Community

In a nutshell, children, parents, network and therapists, as a group, form a (working) community that strives to improve the situation for everyone.

5.3 Children

Attention on the children

No Kids in the Middle revolves around the children – they are central. Being connected with children also implies being connected with parents, families and networks. Parents and other people involved are acknowledged for their good intentions; everyone wants the children to have a good life and a good future.

Attention on the interspace

Children do not suffer so much from living a separated life with their parents, but from the space between the parents: the *interspace* (see section 3.2.2). The space where conflicts dominate care and tasks, transfer, clothes, hairdo, food, rules, school, holidays, money and anniversaries. In fact, everything that touches on the life of children. The space between the parents in conflict is always loaded with tension, anxiety and aggression. The stress placed on the children in the interspace is blamed by the parents on the visit with the other parent. This is how stress in children can again lead to demonizing and escalating conflicts which may, in turn, cause children to feel guilty. We actively present the different interspace-related themes to the children. Then, we follow the children in what they want or don't want to do with the themes.

Listening and taking seriously

Listening to children and taking them seriously means following children. There is room to speak and not to speak, to play or not to play, to be occupied creatively or not. In the group, peer support is encouraged: children can help and support each other. There is attention towards their pain and their resilience.

Empathizing with children, hearing and seeing them also means that there is attention given to the different development phases. Small children have different needs and other responsibilities than adolescents. There is room for these differences.

There is also room for the children's loyalty to their parents. Parents are not being demonized. Therapists are not "the better parents". It may be that children are not ready to open their inner world in a group just yet, when they are still living in a world of conflict and battle. If parents are not (yet) able to reduce the tension, the therapists may also support the children in their "survival strategy" to seclude themselves and to turn their minds to other things, like sports, music and friends.

5.4 Letting go

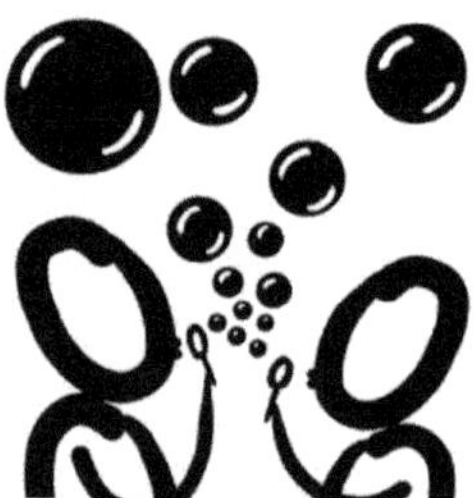

This keystone relates to the desired change process. To make the stress and conflicts decrease, it is essential that parents, children and therapists can let go: let go of each other as ex-partner and the other parent, of the illusion of control and of there being one truth (make room for tolerating ambivalences), and also letting go of the tensions.

Transition to a new stage of life

Parents who remain caught in conflicts do not get separated. A quarrelsome divorce is a failed divorce. The transition from the old situation, whether married and living together or not, to the new situation of letting go of each other and wishing each other the best, has not been completed. Parents remain stuck in an intermediate stage, also called the liminal stage (see section 2.2.6). That has to do with the conviction of parents that the other parent needs to change or leave, and that conviction is mutual. That conviction takes the form of a monologue into which the network is dragged. Parents, often with the support of others, continue to hang on to the illusion of control and think that they can change the other as long as they dedicate themselves enough to it. They cannot bear the tragedy of the differences, of the divorce.

Some of them cannot mourn about the divorce and cannot accept that life is not malleable. It is important that parents forgive each other and resign themselves to their past.

Tolerating ambivalences

Letting go is also connected with being able to tolerate the ambivalence of multiple voices, of differences and multiple truths.

Children, too, need to learn to tolerate ambivalent feelings. It helps them accept that parents are different and live in a different way. That parents are good and loving, but that they have their drawbacks, too, like themselves. Children must learn to deal with the differences in the different houses and the different families. Most children are able to do so as long as these differences are not laden with blame, accusations and demonizing.

Sometimes, children manage to break away from the battle that is going on between their parents and accept the differences between their parents. These are usually older children of secondary school age, who are more independent and have more room to exert their independence.

Small children cannot do this since they are in a dependent relationship. Others can, however, support them to cope with the differences. For them, the transition of the parents needs to precede the transition of the children: when the parents stop their continuous conflicts, the children will be freed.

Illusion of control

Parents often remain caught in the illusion that they can control the other. An example: Chips are nice and unhealthy. That means that you eat chips now and then. In a quarrelsome divorce this becomes the issue in a battle. A child will tell its dad that she ate chips at her mum's: "That's unhealthy, isn't it dad?" Parents tend to use this to strengthen their own conviction that things are not going well at the other parent's house and will not connect it with ambivalence and multiple voices. In this example, the father sends an angry note to the mother stating that she should take better care of their child. The child would learn to tolerate ambivalences if father would say: "That is true, but I think that you enjoyed eating them". For the father to say this, he must let go of the idea of control of the weekends at the mother's house. Children will only have room to tolerate ambivalence if parents can do this.

Therapists, too, must learn to let go of the illusion of control. Therapeutic efforts and commitment do not always lead to the desired change. They have an obligation to perform to the best of their ability, not an obligation to produce a certain result. They create a context which allows for change, but they cannot make sure that this change will actually take place. They do not control it. As Bateson said: "You can take the horse to the water, but you cannot make it drink" (Bateson, 1972). Therapists give their effort and commitment and then have to be able to let go, too. Sometimes, the programme works out well. Sometimes, it doesn't. Sometimes, only later.

In the programme, the therapists, the parents and the network explore what they need to be able to do to let go of the illusion of control together. Then they can shape their own life with their children and other people close to them as best they can, and no longer put energy in changing the other or in trying to control the situation. The treatment programme supports parents in the positive processes, such as accepting, forgiving, letting go, trusting and validating proper parenting.

5.5 Destructive patterns

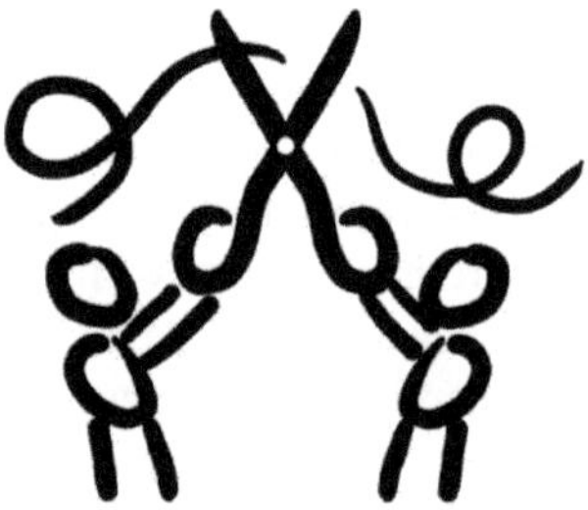

Parents are often caught in destructive patterns of attack and defence. Patterns everyone is drawn into. Therapists recognize and decrease the destructive patterns by connecting them with the vulnerability cycle and working on emotion regulation.

These parents are often shocked and hurt by nasty experiences in their relationship before or during the divorce, or by experiences from earlier relationships or from childhood. Wounds are connected with stress. When old wounds are touched on, stress increases. The higher the stress, the less people can regulate emotions. They enter the survival mode of fight, flight or freeze, and these survival strategies can again trigger the wound of the other. Like the man who retreats and, by doing so, triggers the feeling of the woman, "I am being deserted again". Or, the woman continuously blaming the man and, by doing so, triggers his fear that, again, he does not live up to expectations.

These processes can start a vulnerability cycle which escalates and is hard to break (see Chapter 2, section 2.2). In No Kids in the Middle, there is attention towards these relational processes.

Parents, children and therapists work together to regulate emotions. We acknowledge the wounds and the pain in all parents and children. The therapists validate the feelings that go with these wounds and pain. It is important for the pain and wounds of the parents, but also for grandparents and new partners, relatives and friends.

Social workers and therapists can feel hurt, too, when working with these problems. Attention towards the wounds of the therapists is just as important as attention on the pain of the clients.

Children are also often shocked and hurt by the destructive parental conflicts, or by the one-sided interpretation by parents of the behaviour and the feelings of the children. If a child says, for instance, that the stepfather can be quite strict and the father immediately uses this in the battle with mother, a child may feel guilty. For the child, it would be much better if the father helped find a way to deal with the strict behaviour of the stepfather. Together with the child, the father can emphasize the stepfather's good sides.

By acknowledging and validating wounds and pain, the stress may be reduced. People can think about alternative behaviour again and start to empathize with others again.

It is a basic skill in the No Kids in the Middle programme to recognize stress-induced reactions in the other and oneself and, then, to calm down. If trauma plays a role, these reactions are even more intense and it is even more difficult to regulate emotions.

5.6 Changing by experiencing

Words and insight alone do not bring about change. Experiencing, feeling, living through, acting, creativity and presenting are crucial in the success or otherwise of a change process. The entire human being needs to be involved in such a process. That is why there is a lot of room for experience exercises, assignments and actions in this programme.

Children get the opportunity to talk about relevant topics or not. There is also a lot of room for creativity, moving and acting. The therapists do body-oriented work with the children. Where is stress in your body and how can you move to make it reduce? Children draw and do craftwork about their lives. This may relate to the themes of the children's group (see Chapter 9) or just what they feel like drawing or crafting at some point about what works and about what they find difficult. Children make a presentation for the parents and therapists in which they make them see, hear and feel how it is to be a child of parents who argue a lot. In their presentation, they also incorporate their wishes for the near and far future. Nearly all children incorporate that they would like the conflicts to stop in their presentation. In the children's group, there is also a lot of playing – a ball game, emotion game or another game. This helps children to loosen up while the parents are working hard in another room.

In the programme, parents are invited to put themselves in their children's shoes by doing experience exercises. They sit on children's chairs between battling parents or parents who ignore each other and formulate their thoughts, feelings and physical sensations. In the warm-up (see Chapter 4, section 4.5.2) we do body-oriented exercises with parents and children together.

Parents do homework at home with the people around them (van der Elst et al., in press). Parents, for instance, have to explain the destructive interaction patterns to their network, and how they are caught in these patterns themselves. They learn how they can free themselves, their children and other people involved from these destructive patterns. They watch films about conflict divorces, again with their network.

Parents also make a new, non-demonizing story about separating – a story with which the children can live.

In the discordant period, parents tend to tell the same story repeatedly: we don't live together anymore because the *other* has made it impossible, the *other* is the cause, and the children and I are the victims. Now, too, things are not going well because of misbehaviour by the *other*. Since all parents tell stories with such a plot, children have to live with two conflicting stories. Some children (and most adults) opt for one story, for one parent. Children can also say different things to different parents because they tend to believe parents but get confused by the different stories. Parents are invited to tell their story again and in such a way that the other does *not* get the blame for everything; in a way that the other is left whole and that the other can listen to the story without getting very angry or needing to walk away. A story in which both parents are people with good and bad sides, and are both people who want the best for their children. Those are stories with which children can live, and in which there is room for ambivalence.

At the end of the programme, parents also present what they have learned in the group and what they want for the future for their children, themselves and the people around them.

Chapter 6

Intake and referral

6.1 Referral and contraindication

The screening and matching of care seekers, care providers and interventions is a complex matter. It requires quality at the gate. It means that highly skilled specialists in divorce procedures are needed to perform a proper screening and to weigh when a low-impact intervention is appropriate and when clients should immediately be referred to high-intensity forms of care.

A proper screening at the gate prevents a lot of trouble later on in the process. It is a known fact that people often receive low-impact forms of intervention when they have complex problems. As a result, the intervention fails and clients lose confidence in the care providers. The more complex the problems, the more need for tailoring. When clients are referred to No Kids in the Middle, we therefore also conduct our own screening to find out if our treatment programme meets the needs of these people. And the parents who have been referred to us can consider themselves whether they think that the group intervention suits them or not, and if they would like to join the programme or not.

Assessing referrals is a complex matter, especially for a complex group like parents and children who are caught in a quarrelsome divorce. The stages of conflict are often used to base the assessment on. Divorces, however, only rarely proceed as predictably as the frequently used conflict escalation ladder of Glasl (2001), where conflicts increasingly escalate from stage 1 to stage 7. A break-up may be linked to relational trauma and violence, in which case the conflict may enter the highest stage at once. But a quarrelsome divorce may also fall back into a more peaceful divorce, when both parents have, for instance, found a new partner who take a de-escalating stand.

Client variables form another complicating factor, such as intelligence, educational level, physical and mental health, and whether clients have a supportive social network or not and a sound financial basis (de Van Jonge & Peen, 2013).

Therapist variables, too, play an important role. Some therapists are good at working with groups, while others are overcome by the number of people and perform better with a single client or a couple. Some therapists are good at working with escalating conflicts, others get stressed out by it and, as a result, can no longer work effectively. The main thing is that therapists have affinity, are well-educated and clock up flying hours.

Learning effects are also at play. We have noticed that we have become more effective throughout the years. In more recent groups, families have benefited more from the intervention. We have learned from working with these families and from each other, and we have become increasingly better.

It is therefore not possible to give a clear and uniform answer to the question: Who should be referred to the No Kids in the Middle programme, and when? In the sections that follow, some of the outcomes of our discussions are explained, and they may put you on the right track. They are not strict directions for assessing referrals.

6.1.1 Indications for referral

Duration of the divorce

The programme is intended for parents who have been divorced or separated for more than a year and who are caught up in complex conflict patterns. This is because conflicts after a divorce are normal and are part of a process of separation. It is not helpful to problematize conflicts too soon. Conflicts also help people cope with the painful process of divorce and to get through the liminal stage of the divorce (see section 2.2.6).

Vulnerability of parents and children

Many parents and children who come to us for treatment are vulnerable. They may suffer from traumatic experiences and be easily triggered or suffer from another psychological vulnerability. Parents also accuse each other of psychopathology: "she suffers from borderline personality disorder", "he is a narcissist, a psychopath or an autist". As long as the stress is high between parents or in the children, it is hard to assess whether a parent suffers from psychopathology. De-escalation is needed first.

So, although we do not deny that there are often signs of vulnerabilities, stress reactions and psychopathology, we first aim at de-escalation and increasing safety. If we manage to do so, the fog will lift and we will be much better able to see what problems are still at play. This goes for both the parents and the children. Since we have a lot of experience with working with vulnerabilities and/or psychopathology, this is not a contraindication.

What is needed, however, is a certain measure of emotion regulation for the group treatment to be beneficial. Parents who are easily triggered and cannot properly regulate their emotions get furious, explode, walk away or freeze. That is not good for themselves, but neither for the group process and the children involved. For these parents, a preliminary treatment is needed, for instance, a trauma treatment.

Age of the children

Children from four to 18 years old can participate in the children's group. Children under four have not developed enough socially and cognitively to benefit from therapy in a children's group. For these children, therapy with parents, with attention on the parent-child relationship, is the way to go (see section 6.1.4).

It seems that parents with children between eight and 12 years old benefit most from the therapy. We think that this is because the parent-child relationship is still very strong in this phase: parents see and feel that the children need them. At the same time, children of this age are autonomous enough to let parents know what they think and feel in conflict situations. Because of the combination of dependence and autonomy in the parent-child relationship, parents in these families may be motivated most to change when they start to realize how important the *interspace* is for children.

Still, a large number of children between 12 and 18 have also come out stronger. They benefit most from a combination of group sessions and individual sessions. They are often better able to distance themselves from all conflicts and to focus on their own lives. Children over 18 cannot be referred; the programme falls under youth care. All the same, also young people of 19 and even 21 have followed (part) of the programme, at their own request, when younger brothers or sisters attended, too.

Contact between parents and children

In case of a quarrelsome divorce, children sometimes do not want to see one of their parents. There are many reasons why. It may be that the child in question has had very bad experiences with and memories of that parent, or has witnessed serious incidents of interparental violence. But it can also be that the child is drawn into the parental conflict and has found themselves on one side. Then, the child's reasons for not wanting to see the parent are not consistent with actual experiences of the child itself.

When conflicts drag on, adults usually take sides, too. Although relatives or friends resolve not to take sides, it often proves impossible to maintain contact with both parents. It is also felt as a threat or even as betrayal by one or both parents. For children, too, it is quite a task to maintain relations with both parents while they are in conflict, demonize each other and tell very different stories. It is understandable that children take sides, just like the adults around them do.

It is the task of the parents to create an environment in which it is safe for the child to have contact with both of them. No Kids in the Middle does not aim to restore the contact between parent and child. The goal is to reduce the parental stress so that parents let go of each other and get separated, and that the space between them becomes peaceful and allows the child to have contact with both.

For a child to join No Kids in the Middle, they have to be prepared to come to the group sessions and to see both parents during the break, during the warm-ups at the start of the sessions and during the presentations. We do not force contact, but we do offer the opportunity for contact. Children who refuse to come if the alienated mother or father (both occur) is present cannot enrol. In that case, the entire family is excluded from participation.

Network

If parents cannot or do not want to bring members from their network, this impedes a positive outcome. People in the network around the parent may bring positive change, but may also inhibit it. The network is needed to bring about lasting change together.

In a nutshell, the group intervention No Kids in the Middle is intended for families with parents who have been divorced or separated for more than a year, who are caught up in complex conflict patterns where vulnerabilities are often at play, and who find it hard to regulate their emotions. They must be prepared to reflect on themselves and to involve people from their network in the process. They need to be prepared to stop legal proceedings or to put them on hold. The children must be prepared to come along and to meet both parents at the intervention centre.

6.1.2 Contraindications

It is not possible to participate in No Kids in the Middle:

- If parents do not want to put their court proceedings on hold.
- If parents indicate that they cannot attend all meetings.
- If there is actual physical violence in the relationships.
- In cases of serious addiction to drugs or alcohol. In that case, the person in question will be referred for care and treatment of their addictions first.
- If parents are not able to regulate their emotions, if they explode easily or if they are psychotic.

6.1.3 If a preliminary treatment is indicated

The goal of a preliminary treatment is to create a situation in which the child and the parents may participate in the group programme. Preliminary treatment is offered if the contraindications can be changed.

Vulnerability of parents

During preliminary treatment a parent can learn to deal with emotions, allowing him or her to become part of the group. Some parents are not capable of controlling their emotions enough since they are traumatized. A trauma-centred treatment with exposure and/or EMDR is then suggested first.

Current violence in the family

A treatment is suggested to first permanently stop the violence (see also section 4.3).

Contact between parents and children

Preliminary treatment is suggested if a child does not want to see a parent, even at the treatment centre. The methodology of Asen (2016) may, for instance, be used for the preliminary treatment. His methodology is in line with that of No Kids in the Middle.

6.1.4 No Kids in the Middle for individual families

The programme can be offered to one family only when parents are able to explain why it is impossible for them to join the group, although they are motivated to make the change. For instance, case involving celebrities. We were concerned, too, about the effects if they were to join group sessions. Another example is that of a mother who frequently had to travel abroad for work while the children stayed at their father's house and, for that reason, would be absent a lot.

Too young children

In families with children under four who are excluded because of the children's age, we sometimes have good experiences with following those steps of the programme in which the children and the network, and all other keystones, play a significant role. In these cases, too, it is important to work with two therapists. This will make it a time-consuming and expensive approach, however, which may only be proposed in exceptional cases.

6.2 Referral

Referrals often come via youth and family centres, from child protection services, judges or colleagues, but mediators, GPs and social workers also make referrals to the No Kids in the Middle programme. We have also had word-of-mouth referrals from clients who were pleased with the changes the programme had brought. Usually, referrals are made out of concern for the children. Some children have a variety of complaints. People around them, including professionals, want the complaints to be examined and the child to be treated.

If the referral reveals that there is an ongoing battle between parents not living together, with kids caught in the middle, it is important to explain to parents (and the network) that the context needs to come to rest first. Only then may the child be examined for any remaining problems. Parents and the network can be very persistent in their demand to have the child examined and treated first. However, to go along with that is a malpractice.

There are also children who show (over)adjusted behaviour and never cause any problems; they never want to give rise to conflicts. There are concerns about these children, too, but more often among professionals than among parents.

Sometimes, immediate referrals are made to No Kids in the Middle when specialist care is needed to stop the destructive battle between the parents and to restore a safe environment for the children in which they can develop.

Given that parents in this target group are quick to put the blame for what goes wrong on something other than themselves (on the other parent or social workers), or tend to think that things that go wrong or just happen to them, we place the responsibility and control on the parents from the moment of the registration. We extend the meta-level message to them that if they think that something has to change, they can control it with their own behaviour.

When a referral comes in, the parents are expected to register for the programme themselves by contacting us. Then, we check if parents are eligible for an exploratory talk:

- Is the age of at least one of the children between four and 18?
- Have the parents been divorced or separated for at least one year?
- Does one of the participating children live in the municipality that reimburses for No Kids in the Middle?

As soon as both parents have enrolled and these questions have been answered affirmatively, we will invite them for an exploratory talk.

Only if the parents experience too much stress when being together in one room to properly digest information will we arrange to see the parents separately.

6.3 Exploratory talk with parents

The first talk is with the parents only. Preferably, with the parents together. It is an exploratory and an introductory talk. There will be a substantive intake interview, with the children present, only if the parents decide to join the programme. We do not invite the children earlier, so as not to give them false hope. The first talk lasts 45 minutes and aims to:

- get acquainted;
- provide information about the programme and the method of working;
- provide information about the conditions for participation;
- provide an opportunity for parents to ask questions; and
- decide together whether participation may help improve the problems.

If, already during the meeting, parents decide to enrol, the aim is also to:

- give further details about scientific research and ask them to participate in the research (optional); and
- arrange the paperwork surrounding participation.

The exploratory talk starts with getting acquainted. The therapists of the parent group, and the parents if they want to, tell something about themselves. We explain the goal of the meeting and also that parents can ask questions whenever they want. We explicitly say that we do not go into detail about their problems and conflicts.

We give an explanation of the programme, how it all started, that the children are central, why group sessions can be so effective and how the sessions are structured. We explain that the atmosphere in the groups must allow for a relationship based on trust to develop, and that parents need to make sure that they and their children are always present and come on time. For participants, it inspires confidence when the same people are always there, and that people do not just stay away or rush in late. We also ask parents not to share with their children what has been discussed in the parent group, something which the children wouldn't do either.

We hope to witness parents doing their best for their children in a new way (see also section 4.3). Since parents nearly always go into the interview with a lot of stress, it has a calming effect when therapists first talk about the programme for a while. It has often been a long time since the parents last sat together in one room or were together without tensions and conflicts. While taking in information, they calm down, get used to each other's presence and get to know the therapists a little better. That is why we prefer parents to come together. If this it too high a threshold and parents are so stressed out that they cannot take in information, we can also see them separately. It is not yet a therapeutic talk. Parents do not talk about the battle which they are caught up in. We do ask parents what they want to achieve. Actually, all parents can express in their own words that they want the conflicts to finally stop, that they need peace and quiet, that they want to go on with their lives, that they want "it" to stop. Most parents have already tried a lot to improve the situation, such as mediation, therapy, legal proceedings and other interventions. The fact that both parents want rest and that they want "it" to stop marks the beginning of the de-escalation of the battle.

Many parents have lost heart. They cannot believe that the situation really might improve. They think that the other is the cause of the problems and they feel powerless themselves. The therapists explain that this goes for all parents who sign up for No Kids in the Middle. All parents point at each other and that makes everything stagnate and their children remain caught in the middle. The therapists explain that the No Kids in the Middle approach involves parents getting to work on themselves and finding out what they could do differently themselves to improve the situation. And then they start to realize that it takes a lot of hard work.

We ask a lot from parents. We demand that they bring their network before the group sessions start and that they do assignments at home after each session. We tell them that we cannot change the situation in eight sessions of two hours and that, in particular, a lot needs to be done at home. That is why there is an evening for the network, new partners, grandparents and others, too. We ask them to support the parents and to do the assignments together at home. Parents who join the programme receive a workbook containing all the assignments. The therapists ask if parents are prepared to really commit to what they can change themselves instead of always pointing at the other. Both parents need to say YES to that.

Then, we explain that treatment and legal proceedings do not go together (Groen, 2013). We will ask parents if proceedings are still going on and if they can be stopped or at least be put on hold. This often proves to be a difficult issue. Many parents are still engaged in legal proceedings and do not want to give up on them. In their fears and desperation, they cling to their lawyer who may step into the breach. They are afraid to lose out when they let go of their lawyer and stop the legal proceedings.

In legal proceedings, it is about winning or losing, and that creates distrust. If I say that, it may be used against me, or I have to remember what he just said or even secretly record it with my phone, because it may serve me well in court. In the treatment we ask people to be vulnerable and to work on more trust so that the situation will be safe again for the children. We ask people to reflect on their behaviour, and that means trying out new behaviour and weighing things up without immediately communicating them with the lawyer. We have found that reflecting and being vulnerable does not work when people continue to be engaged in a legal battle.

If both or one of the parents are/is not prepared to stop the proceedings or to put them on hold, they are excluded from the programme. We have once made an exception for a family that expected a decision from the judge two weeks after the start of the programme, under the strict condition that they would not appeal to a higher court and would abide by the judge's decision.

We mention that trainees attend the sessions of the parent and the children's group, write reports and make video recordings. That is not up for discussion. The reports are needed and the video recordings are meant to be used for the treatment. We use parts of them outside the treatment only after having requested and received written consent to do so.

Finally, we ask parents if they can already decide if they want to be part of the programme or if they want to think it over for a while. Sometimes, parents need time to confer with their lawyer to find out if proceedings can be stopped or put on hold. We do ask them, however, to let us know within a week if they will join, for if they don't, another family will be invited. Therapists may also need time to talk things over, for instance when there seems to be very poor emotion regulation, or when there are concerns about addictive behaviour or current violence.

If parents decide they want to enrol and give their consent, we can seek information from the referrers. When therapists have doubts about participation of a certain family, this is discussed in the team and we can decide to arrange for another talk or a preliminary treatment (see also section 6.1 Referral and contraindication).

Many parents get motivated during the explanatory talk or they were already motivated and they confirm right away that they wish to participate. In that case, an intake interview will be scheduled for them and for their children. Before parents are invited to the intake interview, *both* parents must fill out and send in an open questionnaire (see Appendix 1) and arrange for a referral from their GP or via a youth and family centre. We will also ask them if they are willing to participate in scientific research. Finally, we refer to The Intake, *A Workbook for the "No Kids in the Middle" Intervention Programme*, with information about the intake procedure.

6.4 Intake with parents and children

6.4.1 Joint start

We start the intake interview with parents, children, the two parent therapists and one or two of the child therapists. In a short introduction round, we say our names and we mention whether we are going to work with parents or children. We collect the documents (referral letters, etc.). One of the therapists asks the parents' permission to address the children and then says:

> You are in a house where many children, parents and sometimes also grandmothers and grandfathers come together because they worry about something. We try to help them take away these worries. We are very pleased to do so. You have come here for a project called No Kids in the Middle, which is intended for children and their divorced or separated parents, who often disagree. We have found that children do not like that at all. [Usually children start to nod here] But you are lucky, too. Do you know why? . . . Because your parents have come to understand how unpleasant that must be

> for you and they want to do something about it. And not all parents are willing to do that . . . And we have explained that they will have to work very hard to do so, and that they will receive a lot of homework. And they have agreed to do this anyway. Here, parents get homework, the children don't. (Children often smile when they hear this.) You will join a group of children of divorced or separated parents. Now, we are going to talk with your parents and you will go with our colleagues. They will tell you all about the children's group.

Before the children leave, we ask the parents if the children can tell everything they want to tell. Parents always say "yes" to that, even though children feel that they cannot tell everything. Still, it is good for the children that parents give this approval.

6.4.2 The parents

Goal of the intake interview with the parents is:

> Gain insight into the vulnerabilities of both parents and how they reinforce each other in the "vulnerability cycle" (see section 2.2.1).

We explain that all 12 parents taking part in the group have their own story of everything that has happened. That they have evidence, lots of reports, verdicts of the Child Welfare Council, advice from child protection service, practical examples, and many memories to prove that they are right and the other parent is wrong. We explain that it is our experience that if we talk to a father separately, we truly believe that the mother is no good, and vice versa. And we explain that we know by now that both parents have their own truth and their own reality. Often these seem to exclude each other, but they almost always precisely complement each other.

We also explain that, so far, parents have often asked us to stop other parents when they tell their story about everything that has happened because it is so painful to hear and to see, and that it comes to nothing. That parents, however, ask us to stop the other parent and limit their story exactly because it is the other parent's story, and that they would like to have an opportunity themselves to bring the old pain and memories as evidence to prove themselves right. In the group, we see that parents provoke each other with certain behaviour, with remarks, with gestures or with facial expressions, which makes them think right away: "You see? There he/she goes again . . . always the same". This causes the stress to instantly build up, causes a lot of irritation and anxiety, and parents will no longer be able to listen to each other. All parents recognize this immediately when we explain this during the intake.

Not infrequently, part of the problem is related to shocking events and sometimes even to trauma reactions. Since shocking and stressful events may be related to childhood, but also to the relationship, the two therapists each briefly go to another room with one of the parents. There, the parents can talk about shocking events that may have occurred in their lives and the therapists will help them gain insight into their vulnerabilities. These individual talks last about 30 minutes.

The therapist starts with an explanation:

> We would like to understand a little better what is so painful for you, what has shocked you so much. The therapists are going to talk about that later and then you can listen. But first let me ask you what has moved or shocked you so much. In the period of the divorce, before that in the relationship, or maybe in previous relationships or in your childhood. If I ask what shocked you so much, what comes to your mind?

Parents then tell, for instance, about the shock that the other turned out to be in a relationship with someone else for some time already and had been lying about that the entire time. Or that the other seemed to be very caring at first, but later appeared to be very egoistic and was never at home, or got very furious and even violent in conflicts. Where possible, the therapists link the shocking events to other painful events in life, like the father who was never there or the mother with her fits of rage. People link painful experiences to their self-image. For instance: "You see, I am worthless". They can react to that by withdrawing themselves, or, on the contrary, by showing that they are worth it.

We also ask how the relationship started. Was it a good time, had they really been in love and what was so attractive about the other? We also comment about how sad it is that it can go so terribly wrong anyway. We ask these questions to form a picture. It is not about treatment and we will not go into detail. The interview will focus in particular on what behaviour of the other parent causes stress and triggers negative thoughts about the other parent, but often also about him/herself. We show understanding for reactions to stress or trauma and how difficult it can be to be with the other parent in one room, for instance when there has been violence in the relationship. When there is trauma, we ask questions about care. We will point out that we will deal with the subject of stress and trauma reactions in the group, since this is something that many parents go through.

At the end, we ask if anything new has been said – something which the other did not already know. Usually, this is not the case. Only rarely does a parent not want the therapist to share something in the subsequent joint discussion. Usually, everything can be shared.

Back together, the therapists report on the two brief talks and what they have understood about the start of the relationship and about what has been so painful when things went wrong. They do so in a searching manner. They search for common grounds in the stories, where the stories reinforce each other and how this often painful process evokes destructive patterns. While talking about this, they formulate hypotheses. This is done in the presence of the parents. The therapists describe a vulnerability cycle between the parents in which they reinforce each other's behaviour and in which they are caught.

After the reflections of the therapists, the talk is over and the children are invited in. It is striking to see that after the reflections by the therapists, parents are usually very calm, they feel recognized and heard, and they go home with a new perspective.

It is our experience that many parents are fighting a fierce battle about violence that has or has not taken place. Often, both parents accuse each other of the use of physical, sexual and/or emotional violence. Since the therapists do not know if this has really taken place or if it is part of the fierce battle in which anything can be used as a weapon, they point out that establishing the truth is, of course, important, but that all truths need to be accommodated. The therapists explain that the treatment is about reducing stress levels and increasing safety. And that, in doing so, the children are central.

Any traumas and other painful experiences with the partner can be dealt with in their own network, together with relatives, friends or their own therapist. The relationship with the partner has come to an end, so there is no space for dealing with that with the ex-partner. We focus on "good enough" parenting, and we understand that it is not easy to work together with the other parent if shocking events have taken place, but that it is truly necessary if they both want to be a parent.

There is attention given to accusations about violence towards children. If one of the parents says that the other parent uses physical or sexual violence, then, obviously, this will not be ignored. If reports of violence date back quite some time and have not been declared plausible or risky by the youth and family centres involved, then we will pay attention to it, but the group programme will be our priority.

If there appears to be new information or if one or both parents feel(s) unsafe, then we will pay attention to that before the parents join the group. If this information emerges during the treatment, then a separate talk may be scheduled in between sessions.

The team of four therapists, two of the parent group and two of the children's group, will confer about a possible next step to guarantee the safety of the children (and obviously of the parents, too). Being able to recognize signs in children is very important. This is a very complex area, considering that in many quarrelsome divorces, accusations of violence and neglect by the other parent are part of the battle. But this cannot be a justification for letting safety fade into the background, because the group therapy aims at reducing tensions between the parents. The therapists frequently need to confer and, considering all the care provided before, weigh the steps to be taken as best they can (see also section 4.3). The therapists will go through the dates and conditions and will once again stress that it is important that everyone is present at all sessions.

Finally, the therapists explain that the programme starts with an information evening for all parents and their networks. This evening session is the start of the treatment and is compulsory. We explain how the evening will proceed. If desired, we can help parents think of possible people in their network to bring along to the evening session, with a guideline of two to five people from their network. New partners and grandparents are especially welcome, but also friends and other people involved. These should be people from the network who are important for the children and who are part of the battle or, on the contrary, have managed to stay out of it so far.

6.4.3 The children

Some children like to come and want to talk about how things are at home, while some children are reluctant to talk. Children have often noticed that anything they say can be used as ammunition in the battle between the parents and they have learned to stay quiet and not to commit themselves. For each child, we try to find out what works. Sometimes, we work a lot with a ball and we do not talk much. Sometimes, we talk a lot. What follows is a list of questions the therapists may ask, which may vary for each child. We always start with an introductory game with a ball. During the game or afterwards, we give information about the talk and about the group.

Goal of the talk with the children:

- Get acquainted with children and therapists.
- Provide information to the children about the group.
- Provide an opportunity for the children to ask questions about the group.
- A first exploration of what the *interspace* does to the children.
- Give the children a voice: on what points are the children doing fine? What is their strength? What do they worry about? Which situations do they find hard to deal with and what do they find difficult? What works? Who can they turn to for support?

The children's therapist explains the goal of the talk:

> We will get to know each other a little better, ask some questions and explain what we are going to do in the group.

The children's therapists will give details about the groups:

> Your family is going to participate in No Kids in the Middle, together with five other families. All parents come together in one group and so do the children. This makes for one parent group and one children's group. All parents of these families live apart. Some are divorced or separated, and some have never lived together, but they do have children together, of course. And in all cases, parents find it hard to deal with each other and to confer about their children in a peaceful and friendly way, and their children may suffer from that. They feel the tensions, and sometimes read messages or hear parents talk about each other in a nasty way. It gives some children a headache or a stomach ache. Others sometimes feel very much alone. Each child may suffer from it in a different way. There are also children who do not suffer much from it. But, fortunately, your parents want to learn to deal with each other in a better, friendlier and more relaxed way. That is why they go to the parent group. Nobody knows for sure if they will succeed, but it is nice to know that they at least want to try. And, of course, your parents also do things well. We would like to hear about that, too. All six families come together on the same day and at the same time, once every two weeks. Your parents will tell you on which days you will come. In total, you will come eight times to the group.

> All parents and children wait together in the family room until we, the therapists, invite you to your room. Then, all parents, children and therapists start together in the parent group and we will do something nice. Sometimes we sing, we blow bubbles or we do something else. After that, the children go to their own room. In the children's group, you will talk, draw, craft and do many other things. In each session, we will also talk about how it is to be a child of parents living apart and who find it hard to be nice to each other. You may also help each other by giving tips. In the group, there is one very important rule: You can talk, but you don't have to! The first time you will come to the group is: . . day, from . . . to . . . o'clock.

The therapists explain that it is about reducing the tensions between the parents, so that the children suffer less from the tensions and may start to feel better. They will do things in the group they like to do, such as making photos and videos, drawing, graffiti, music, dance and other activities about topics which children find important when their parents do not live together. Children can ask questions and say what they think of the idea.

The child therapists explain:

> We have already talked with a lot of children whose parents are divorced or separated and continue to argue. Most children suffer from that, because it causes tensions and children often don't know where they stand. We are going to ask you a lot of questions, but you only need to answer if you want to. You can also say "I don't know". And you may also want to tell something without us asking about it. You can do so anytime. You may ask us any question anytime. For instance, why we want to know something. You may also say that you prefer not to talk about something. We will ask you why not, though, because you come to the group for a good reason. So, you can tell everything. We will not pass anything on to your parents, because what you say here is private. Obviously, there are exceptions. Sometimes, children tell us things which we think parents really should know about. For instance, when it comes to your safety or that of your parents. But we will always confer with you first. Then, we will ask if your father or mother already knows about what you told us and who may know about it, or how we can tell parents about it, for instance together with you or without you. And we discuss what details we think are important to share with parents and we ask you how we may tell your parents.

At the same time, the child therapists and the children will get to know each other a little better in a relaxed way. For instance, by bouncing a ball to each other and asking questions: "What is your favourite colour? Do you have a pet?" Children may also ask questions to the therapists. Often, they ask neutral questions: "Do you like pizza?" or "Do you do sports?" But sometimes, children can also ask confronting questions like: "Are you divorced?" or "Are your parents divorced?" It works best to briefly and honestly answer these questions. The questions of the therapists may gradually move on to the home situation. For instance, if a dog has been mentioned: "Can you bring your dog to dad's house, too?" Gradually, we will start asking specific questions about the home situation.

6.4.3.1 Home and the interspace

The therapists take two large sheets of paper (flip-chart).

> With whom do you live where?

The child therapists explain the following to the children:

> What you see here are two houses (draw them on a large sheet of paper) and we are very curious to know who lives there. Which house is dad's and which house is mum's? If you want, you may colour the houses while we talk. I am going to ask you some questions about it and I will write the answers next to it. Who lives in the house with dad and who lives in the house with mum? Does your dad or mum have a new partner? And are there stepbrothers or stepsisters, or maybe even half-brothers or half-sisters? And do you have pets? What do you like about being with mum? What do you like about being with dad?

GOING FROM ONE HOUSE TO THE OTHER

The therapists ask questions like:

- In which house are you when?
- Are there fixed agreements about that?
- How do you go from one house to the other?
- Does anyone come to get you or take you to the other house. If so, who?

- Do you do any sports during the weekend and are there agreements with your parents about who takes you there and who comes to watch a match?

ARRANGEMENT(S) CONCERNING PARENTAL ACCESS

> Some children may choose where they spend the weekend and they appreciate that very much. Others may also choose, but they don't like that at all, because they do not want to disappoint one of the parents or because they feel guilty if they say what they want. These children just like it when the parents determine where they will spend which days and how often. How is that in your situation?

- Do you ever talk about that with anyone?
- Do you know if both of your parents feel happy about the parental access arrangements?
- Or, does one of your parents want to change the arrangements?
- If so, how does that make you feel?
- Do you feel you can say anything you want about the arrangements?

And when you arrive at the other parent:

- Does your parent step outside the car to see if you are already there?
- Does you parent honk the horn or walk with you to the door to ring the doorbell?
- Do mum and dad talk to each other or don't they?
- Can you describe how things go when a parent comes to get you?
- What do you think about how they deal with that?
- How does that make you feel?

BELONGINGS

- How are your belongings?
- Do you have to pack and take your clothes and stuff every time you go to the other house, or do you have clothes, soft toys and other toys, sporting clothes and gear, and so on in both houses?
- If you have to take your stuff from one parent to the other, do you have to think of that yourself or does someone else pack your things for you, or do you do that together?
- If you have forgotten something, would that be a problem or not? How is that solved or would that be your problem?

- Is it important in one or both houses who pays for your things?
- Do you know who pays for your belongings or is that not at all important?
- If it is important, how do you tell?
- Does that bother you?
- Can you decide about your own things, like what you want and whether you take your things with you or not?

DIFFERENCES AND SIMILARITIES IN BOTH HOUSES

- What is the same and what is different in both houses?
- What rules and agreements are there in both houses?
- Do you have a say in that?
- How do you feel about that?
- Would you like that to change?
- What is very nice in one house and what about in the other?
- What is very annoying or unpleasant in one house and what about in the other?
- Who punishes you when you do something that isn't allowed and who comforts you?
- Where can you laugh and where can you *cry* a lot if you want to?
- Are you okay with how things go now or would you like things to be different?
- And with whom can you talk about that?

For very young children, think of rules about eating, bed times, tidying up and differences in activities. For older children, think of differences in atmosphere.

- How is that for the children? Do the differences bother them or not?
- Are they allowed to call the other parent or not?

How children deal with the differences:

- Do they need time to get used to the situation at the other parent's house?
- How is it for them to go from one parent to the other?
- Do they notice in themselves that they are already thinking about going back to the other parent by the end of the day or, for instance, in the car?

- How is the transfer now and are they comfortable with that?
- Do parents know that?

How do your parents communicate with each other? The following questions will be asked:

- Do your parents have contact with each other?
- In what way do they have contact (by phone, email, WhatsApp, and so on)?
- How do you feel about that?

For children who do not go to one of their parents:

- Can you tell us how that has come about?
- For how long have you not had any contact?
- How do you feel about not having any contact (advantages and disadvantages)?

Contact with new partners, step or half-brothers and sisters, relatives and friends of parents:

- Does one of your parents have a new girlfriend or boyfriend?
- How do you get along with your father's or mother's new girlfriend or boyfriend?
- Does he or she also set rules or agreements?
- What do you really like or don't like about him or her?
- How is that with step and half-brothers and sisters?
- How often are they at home with you?
- Do you have contact with both of your grandfathers and grandmothers?
- Do you have contact with other relatives of both parents, and do they have contact with each other?
- Who talks nice or loving about father/mother and who doesn't?
- Do you have contact with the relatives of you stepfamily, too? Sometimes, children also have a grandfather, a grandmother or other relatives in that family.

DIFFICULT SITUATIONS

> Children often tell us that holidays and birthdays may be difficult situations for them. And that is unpleasant for them, because these are days

they would normally be looking forward to. Or information evenings or performances at school. Or, for instance, taking the final swimming test.

- How is that in your situation?
- How does that make you feel?
- Do you sometimes have to cry about the divorce or the arguments when you are on your own?
- Who can you turn to talk about the situation? Who can support you?
- Who knows that you are having a hard time sometimes?

The questions are examples for conversations with the children. It is not at all necessary to ask all the questions. It should not become a question-answer session. It is important for children to feel that there is room to talk or just say nothing. This makes for a light atmosphere without any pressure. In the first session of the children's group, we deal with the subject in greater detail.

WHAT ARE YOU GOOD AT AND WHAT IS DIFFICULT FOR YOU?

Briefly talk with the children about what they are good at and what they find difficult. Make a connection to the divorce. What are disadvantages and what are advantages of having divorced parents? If possible, ask: Do they have bad memories of the divorce or the period before or after it? Do they have memories of arguments? Check for anxieties, gloominess, sleeping and reliving events. Children's answers and drawings will not be shown to the parents.

Since battling parents make for an unsafe environment for children, we are very careful about sharing information with parents. The most important thing is that children feel heard and seen by the therapists – that they are taken seriously and feel safe with the therapists. Finally, we explain to the children that they can also help each other deal with parents having tensions and give each other tips.

6.5 Group composition

If there are six suitable parent couples, the group will be put together. The strength of the group composition is its diversity (see section 3.2.1).

In addition to diversity in educational background, parents also have different cultural backgrounds. In the groups we have worked with there were a lot of parents with a Dutch cultural background, but also parents from South America, Africa, Poland and Italy. These parents didn't speak Dutch well, but their Dutch was good enough to participate with help from the group. Dutch parents with a Turkish or Moroccan background have also taken part in the programme. Usually, the parents are a father and a mother, but sometimes the parents are two fighting mothers.

Parental age ranges between 35 and 55, and all parents have one or more children under 18. The variation in age is no problem at all. On the contrary, diversity turns out to enrich the group. Where highly educated people are often gifted speakers who tend to beat about the bush, low-educated parents can be very direct, saying for instance: "If you ask me, you are being pretty much concerned about yourself". Parents who do not always quite understand Dutch are helped by Dutch-speaking parents, who are forced to speak clearly and simply because of this language deficiency. In this way, they help both themselves and the other group members.

The diversity makes for a versatile view of fatherhood and motherhood, of family relationships and of the divorce context. This diversity raises relevant questions and breaks through tunnel visions and monologues. The binding factor is the fact that all parents are caught up in discordant and complex divorce processes, in which the care for the children has become one of the main issues of the battle.

There is a small chance that parents know each other. In small communities, chances are higher that this will happen. This is a problem that applies to groups in general, not just to this programme. Fortunately, so far we have not had any case of people joining the programme who turned out to know each other.

Chapter 7

The network meeting

Prior to the group sessions, there will be an information meeting for the parents and their networks at seven in the evening. The children are not invited. This evening is mandatory and is part of the programme.

The network meeting was set up after it turned out that the social network of the parents plays an important role in the course of the divorce and the corresponding complexities as described in the theoretical introduction (see section 2.2.2). It is not two people but two networks that are separating, with relatives, grandparents, new partners, relatives and children of the new partner, friends, neighbours, contacts at school and work, social workers, lawyers and mediators.

If the social network is not aware of the purpose and the goals of the treatment, they tend to comment critically and be unfavourably disposed towards positive steps made by parents in the group. They do so out of concern for the parent they have contact with because they do not trust the new steps and are afraid that their partner, son, daughter, grandchildren or client will be hurt again.

The network must also learn that there is a new point of departure, with a minimal level of trust where small steps, aimed at conciliation, need to be taken to build on this trust as a parent couple. If the battle has been going on for a long time already, many people have become involved and have taken positions. Distrust has grown and drives the actions. Only if there is room for new perspectives and new behaviour again can children be released from the trap they are caught in.

To facilitate cooperation with the networks, we invite the parents and other people who are important to them to the information evening without their children. We aim, in particular, at their private network of relatives and friends, but sometimes parents arrive with their lawyer or social worker. It is not therapy, it is an information evening, like the ones held at school.

A few days before the information evening, we call all parents to ask them with how many people they will bring. This is really necessary to make sure that all the parents will be there with a part of their network. This evening proves to be an important and effective ingredient of the programme.

On the evening itself, the programme is explained as clearly as possible. This includes the background and the method, lively anonymized examples and, optionally, visual material. All therapists are present, including the therapists of the parent group and the therapists of the children's group. It is an information evening in auditorium style. There is *no* introduction round. Only the therapists will introduce themselves. The therapists talk about the parent group and the children's group. They explain that we ask parents to work to change themselves and to step out of the battle, and that this is only possible with the help of the network. We explain that there will be homework assignments, which the parents will get and are supposed to do with people from the network.

The people present at the meeting may ask questions. The therapists will not go into specific examples. One of the attendants asks, for instance: "What if another parent does not want to cooperate?" A possible answer could be:

> Perhaps, right now, you cannot imagine yet that it can really become better. Several of you in this room will have lost hope, but we know that it is possible. We have to, because the children need it. But so do the parents and all of you.

This energy creates new hope, which is needed for the children, the parents and their networks. But the therapists also make clear that success is not guaranteed, and that it doesn't always succeed. If someone asks what happens if it doesn't succeed, we explain that we are always willing to think with them about how to move forward and what other help may be needed in that case.

Apart from the therapists, young experience experts are always present at the information evening. They talk about their experiences as children of divorced parents in conflict. Parents may ask them questions, also anonymously. The questions go into a hat that is passed round. The young people try to answer the questions as best as they can. The contribution of these young people often leaves a deep impression with the parents and the people from their network.

Finally, the therapists ask a very important question to all those present:

> Can you please help us? Without your help, we cannot do it!

We ask the network if they are prepared to come back once again during or after the therapy. We explain that the children need them badly, especially in moments when parents threaten to get stuck in their battle. In this way, we hope to encourage relatives, new partners and friends to cooperate with us and to encourage their loved ones to get moving instead of staying caught in the current impasse.

We have noticed that calling in the network, also later on in the treatment, may well break the impasse between parents. Sometimes, there is an extra session with a grandparent or with a parent of the new partner, sometimes both networks without the parents, sometimes a network of one parent with a parent, and so on. By continually asking the network what move is needed and how they can support that with the children in mind, they can contribute to positive changes.

Chapter 8

The parent group

8.1 Dynamics in the parent and children's group

The goal of No Kids in the Middle is for children to experience less stress in their lives as a result of parents having less conflicts. At the heart of the No Kids in the Middle programme is the therapeutic process in the parent group.

Many children are signed up for therapy with a wide variety of symptoms. Experience has shown that giving therapy to children only may adversely affect the child if the parents are still caught up in their battle. This is partly because the child can experience the therapist as an additional party. When at the father's house, it is difficult for the child to talk about mother and vice versa. The therapist encourages the child to talk about both parents, and that may be confusing. Since the children talk with the therapist about both parents and the problems they experience, they may start to hope and sometimes expect that the therapist will make sure that the problems will be solved, and the therapist cannot do that. This, too, can be confusing.

Another reason is that it may be an effective survival strategy for children not to dwell too much on their feelings when their parents are still fighting. The child protects themselves by not feeling too much and by turning their thoughts to other things. Therapy, on the other hand, directly appeals to the emotional life with questions like: "What do you experience?", "What do you feel?" and "What do you think?" The child becomes more aware of their feelings and feels more (negative) emotions, whereas there is no room yet to cope with these feelings. In these situations, the child is less protected against stress.

Children often cannot talk about their feelings about the divorce or the interspace when they are at home. When they talk about their grief with their father, for instance, he may use that as ammunition in the battle with the mother, and vice versa.

That is why the focus of the programme is on the parents. They have to work hard to create a better environment for their children.

The concept of the parallel parent and children's group provides more safety for the children. As soon as parents start to argue less or are less stressed out, they become more emotionally available for the children. Children feel free and safe to explore and express their feelings, both in the children's group and when they are at their father's and mother's house. Some children already start to feel more room when they see that parents are doing their best.

8.2 Session breakdown

The breakdown of each session of the parent group is as follows:

- warm-up;
- review homework;
- themes and issues;
- break;
- themes and issues (continuation);
- get moving: home assignments; and
- closing words.

Warm-up

The goal of the warm-up is to do something nice with parents and children together to create a positive vibe. We do exercises that match the theme of the children's group. Each session (except for session 6 and 7, in which children and parents show their presentations) starts with parents and children together in the room of the parent group. We chose the parent room since it allows children to see where parents are working to make things better for them. If another room is more suitable, then that is, of course, also fine. The joint start is a warm-up for the main themes that will come up in the children's group. For each session, we will give one or more suggestions for a warm-up. Obviously, there are more possibilities for a warm-up. The joint start appears to work well for both the children and the parents.

Themes and issues

The first three sessions each have a central theme. Each theme includes the following parts:

- information and explanation;
- exercise allowing parents to experience the theme on an emotional and physical level; and
- reactions and questions from parents.

From session 4 on we work on issues that parents keep getting caught up in and for which we will seek new ways with the help of the group. We quite often see that the same themes are an issue in both the parent and the children's group. When, for instance, in the parent group we talk about the pain of missing a child when it is at the other parent's house, in the children's group, the child appears to miss their parents, too.

Break

During the break, the therapists of the children's group and of the parent group come together to update each other and to coordinate things (see section 4.5.1).

Closing words

The therapists close each session by asking each parent to say one word that covers the way they feel when they leave after the session. This gives the parents the opportunity to really round off the session, to briefly reflect on the session and to share a little about how they leave. Words that are often mentioned are: "confusion", "hope", "doubt", "curious", "don't know", "recognition", and "yes and no".

It provides the therapists with some information about how the session has been experienced, how the group members will leave the session and what issues need further attention. The therapists themselves, too, share a final word. For instance: "hope", "connection", or "brave".

8.3 The sessions

The following is a description of sessions 1 to 8.

Session 1

Warm-up

Today, the theme in the children's group is:

> *Getting acquainted and the two houses and the interspace*

The parents sit down on the chairs. The children sit down in front of their parents, on the floor or on a cushion, so that everyone can see which children belong to which parents. This enables the children to see and feel that parents are *behind* the children together. The children do not need to choose whom they are going to sit in front of, their dad or mum. This arrangement also has its effect in the parent group. Parents often keep sitting side by side when the children leave for the children's room. Parents rarely choose this position of their own accord, but by using this arrangement, we give them the feeling that they can stand behind the children and be there for them together – and it shows that we think that they can really do it. Also, in the parent group, we see that this works well.

We do a ball game to get to know everyone's names. We make two circles. The inner circle with children, the outer circle with parents. One of the child therapists steps inside the children's circle and explains that she will pass the ball to the child next to her while saying her name: "I am Margreet". The child next to her does the same with the child sitting next to him or her. After all children have said their name, the ball goes to the first parent. He will introduce himself by saying: "I am John, Kelly's and Kevin's father". After the ball has been passed to all parents and the therapists, you can do another round by throwing the ball to someone you know and, at the same time, saying the person's name. Or, you can throw the ball to someone you do not know and ask for his or her name. Keep the exercise short: no longer than ten minutes the first time.

Other introductory games are:

- Active game: Everyone says their name and, at the same time, does some kind of move. Then, everyone in turn mentions the name of another child who then copies that move. After that, the entire group once again does the move and says the name together.
- "I go to the group and pack my bag", which is similar to the memory game "I pack my suitcase". The first child says the name of the child sitting to the right of him and his own name. The child next to him repeats these names and adds their own name. The last child in the circle says all the names. You can do this one more time. First, with the children's names, and then with the parents' names.

After the warm-up, the child therapists take the children to the children's room.

Welcome

The therapists once again welcome the parents and recognize them for their courage to participate in this programme. It shows that they will do a lot for their children.

One of the therapists briefly introduces the session breakdown:

- 50 minutes of working;
- a fifteen-minute break, which parents and children will have together, while the therapists sit together to confer during the break; and
- 45 minutes of working.

In the beginning, there is not much room for discussion. Instead, the focus will be on getting acquainted and giving information. In this way, parents can listen, quietly observe each other, get used to the fact that they are in the same room with their ex-partner again and the stress in the parents can ease a bit. If one of the parents has a short question, the therapists may briefly go into that.

Since many parents are anxious in the beginning, a lot of questions stem from distrust. Answering these questions alone may increase stress in the beginning. The therapists, on the other hand, aim at reducing stress in the first session. Questions will therefore be positively identified as questions that were raised out of concern for the children. The therapists will say that they have heard the questions, but that the questions will not be dealt with in this phase of the treatment.

We, once again, explain:

- what the children are going to do;
- that the therapists will make sure that all children will be addressed in a way that matches their age and development level;
- that there are always two counsellors (therapists) present and usually also a trainee, to allow for both group and individual work;
- that the children are not in therapy; and
- that most of the work done by the parents is meant to bring about change.

We also explain more about the breakdown of the programme and the presentations the parents are going to give to their children and vice versa.

Getting acquainted

The therapists give the following assignment:

> We would like you to introduce yourself to each other as parents, because the children are central in this programme. You will do so as follows. Everyone briefly shares a short, and preferably recent, memory of each child – a positive moment when you felt connected with that child. It should be something specific, like baking cookies, a chat, playing around or a beach walk. Anything can give us an impression of your relationship. Who wants to start?

The therapists help the parents stick to the assignment. There is a good chance that one of the parents takes this as an opportunity to say that he cannot think of one moment because he has not seen his daughter for two years. The therapists will kindly respond, with attention (present):

> That must be very painful for you, but you surely must have one memory of the time before that which gives us an impression of your relationship with your child(ren).

The therapists listen attentively to the stories. Most of the time, the stories are very short, about a minute per child. If parents start to elaborate, the therapist will help them keep it short. If there are 12 children (two per parent couple on average), then there will be 24 stories. Together, this makes for approximately half an hour. After all 12 parents have told something about the relationship with their child(ren), one of the therapists takes the next step.

For instance:

> What beautiful children, what moving stories, what extraordinary relationships and what a group of parents you are, showing so much love for your children. How terrible that all these beautiful memories have turned into such a painful experience, full of conflict. It is worth a lot to work on that in this group, to create room for all the good you shared with us. After the break, we will explain how something so beautiful can fall apart so badly. We will have a break first. During the break, the therapists sit together and we would like to ask you as parents to make sure that the children do not run around the building. Colleagues are at work in the building. Drinks and fruit are available in the break room. In 15 minutes, we will resume the session.

Explanation of destructive communication patterns

After the break, one of the therapists explains the destructive patterns that are the enemy of family relationships and love relationships. In a simple way, the therapist explains that there are three basic patterns that people can get caught up in and which make their relationship and situation increasingly unsafe and hopeless (see also Figure 8.1):

- the first pattern: approaching – averting;
- the second pattern: approaching – approaching; and
- the third pattern: averting – averting.

An example:

> A approaches B by email, phone or in person, and wants to make something clear to B. A wants, for instance, that B pays closer attention to the gluten-free diet as Tommy always suffers from stomach ache after having been at B's. If the relationship is good, B will listen to this, reassure A and thank A for showing concern. If, however, parents are in a battle, B will either avert and not react or strike back: "You are way too much involved with Tommy with all your rules, it gives him a stomach ache. I can't stand it either. I am glad I don't have to suffer from that anymore. When he is at my place, he never complains about a stomach ache" and so on.

Approaching – averting

In this case, A will not feel heard and will once again try to reach B with the message. This may, eventually, lead to an ongoing argument on the phone or by email. The more A tries to reach B, the more B holds off. B will gradually build a relational wall and will end up turning off the phone.

Approaching – approaching

In this case, there will be blaming back and forth. A wants to make something clear to B and convince B, while B tries to make something clear to A and wants to convince A of being right. And because neither A nor B feels heard, recognized and understood, the blaming will become more intense and corresponding emotions will be more and more desperate. These patterns escalate. We will return to that in session 3.

Averting – averting

The last pattern is that A gives up and no longer tries to get in touch with B, and B also holds off and hides behind a wall. Both lock themselves up in their own defensive tower and in their own truth in which the other person is the perpetrator and the person him/herself is the victim.

While one of the therapists explains these patterns, he draws the patterns as illustrated in Figure 8.1 on the flip-chart. Next, he explains that it is not just the parents that are trapped in the destructive pattern, but that the children get caught in it, too. They are caught in the middle and there is no way out for them. And often, all the other people involved get caught up in these spirals too, even therapists. These destructive patterns draw in more and more people.

Questions can be asked. If someone reacts with an example in which the other parent shows this very behaviour, one of the therapists kindly labels this as a step forward. Everyone joins in and may give examples. The challenge for all parents is to finally give an example of how they act themselves in the pattern. It is easier to see what the other does, but these patterns merely exist by the grace of two parties taking a position. The therapists try to make the parents see how their conflicts keep recurring, not because this theory reveals the truth, but because this way of thinking provides an opportunity for change.

The therapists value all of the reactions of the parents as attempts to cooperate and to think along with them, even though it seems they are

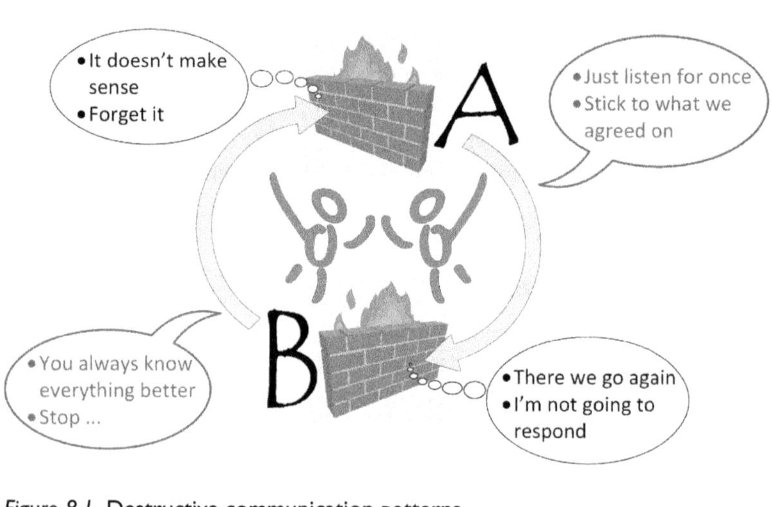

Figure 8.1 Destructive communication patterns

accusing the other instead of looking at themselves: “Very good, you start to recognize it. Are you more on the A or on the B side then?” After all, this is only the first session. With each intervention, you want to open up and identify the field of possibilities. And here this is done by reflecting on own behaviour.

Exercise destructive patterns

Goal

Set parents to work by having them apply the theory about destructive communication patterns to their own situation. Parents will gain insight into how the patterns work in practice. They learn to observe the patterns and to identify them. First in general, then in each other and finally in themselves.

Instruction

> You will break into two groups with a mix of men and women. No parent couples in the same group. Try to find out as a group how to work this out. You will discuss in the group what you recognize from the patterns we just discussed. What do you recognize in yourself, in the other parent and maybe even in another group member? What kind of sentences and/or actions match with these patterns?

Execution

The therapists each join a subgroup and encourage the parents to talk about it with each other. The therapist writes down sentences expressed by the parents: “I cannot keep on answering the phone; it will make my life a misery. I just have to block her phone number”. Another parent may then say: “But if you just pick up the phone and answer, then it would be over, too, wouldn’t it? It’s the same with me. If I don’t know where I stand, then I keep on calling”. After approximately 15 minutes, parents come back to the main group. The therapists reflect in the group on what has come up in the subgroups. They share their observations, considerations, what struck them, what they admire or what worries them. The therapists also mention the pain that goes with the recurring patterns, and they always share what has made them curious and, in so doing, they open up the field of possibilities again for all group members.

Points of interest

In the subgroup, parents often want to grasp the opportunity to explain how impossible the other parent is and how they suffer under him or her, and that the other person obviously suffers from psychopathology and that the other damages the children. The therapist helps to link everything that is said to the destructive patterns. The parents help each other in doing so, too.

The therapist explains that it is not her intention to question the diagnosis of psychopathology or the existence of vulnerabilities as a result of painful events. Experience has shown that it is important to recognize the destructive patterns and to be able to stop them because they cause a lot of stress. When stress starts to decrease, symptoms may also decrease or go away entirely, which is also true in children. That is why the programme starts with recognizing and changing the destructive patterns.

The therapists will keep an attitude of kind presence and will not let themselves be lured into discussions and arguments. Sometimes, this is quite a tall order. That is why it helps to focus on destructive patterns as the common enemy.

Get moving

The therapists briefly explain the home assignment for the second session. See *A Workbook for the "No Kids in the Middle" Intervention Programme.*[1]

Closing words

The therapists close each session by asking all parents to say one word that covers how they will go home after the session.

Session 2

Warm-up

Today, the theme in the children's group is:

> *A house with both parents: how did it start between your parents and what was nice?*

Parents and children are going to blow bubbles together. The exercise is fun, it controls the breathing and it is an easy way to relax. Briefly explain before or after the exercise that blowing bubbles helps to calm the breathing down and to relax.

Make sure that each child has a bottle of bubbles. The children may first blow as many bubbles as they can in one blow. Then, they can give the bottle to one of the parents and blow bubbles together. They can also try to blow as large a bubble as possible. Do this for no longer than five minutes.

Other exercises in which doing fun things together plays an important role:

- One parent drums a beat and everyone copies that beat. This is also something that almost everybody likes to do. Besides, it is an exercise where parents and children need to tune in to one another.
- Singing a song. Singing, too, makes for an even breathing and eases the tension.

Reviewing homework

After the warm-up, we go round the circle and the parents can say if they have got round to doing the home assignments and with whom they have done them. They also share if they have been able to explain to someone in their network how destructive patterns work and if they recognize the patterns in their own situation. Have they been able to do things differently in order to make the patterns less active? Has the other parent noticed that? And the children? How did the network react? We also ask if they have watched the documentary. All parents get an opportunity to answer the questions. It is impossible to predict how this exchange will go.

In a group, a woman said that the documentary by a Dutch celebrity about his HCD parents had really gotten to her. That, when watching the angry father, she had understood the anger of her ex better and that it had made her realize what she had done by choosing another man. Her ex, Paul, was greatly moved by her words; "It is the first time that you acknowledge that", he said. Others said that not only they but also people in their network had recognized the destructive patterns in their own lives and how that had led to a very good and intimate conversation.

In one of the groups, a father immediately starts expressing how unsafe he feels because the mother does not hand over the children when he picks them up and how her boyfriend always opens the door and sends him away. And if he gets angry, they call 112 and report domestic violence. He says that he stays calm now, but that he feels very unsafe. In addition, he often doesn't get to see his children. The mother bursts out with her story about how he had wanted to pull an ill and feverish child out of her arms, and that he had no consideration whatsoever for what is good for the child. The therapist ends the discussion and asks if they recognize which destructive pattern they are caught in now, which is preventing them from listening and which makes them both think that they and the children are treated unjustly. Group members will help and can point out that the parents keep blaming each other without listening to each other.

Often, there is a parent who says: "I recognize all of it. It is the same with me. She always knows better. Women always think that we cannot take care of a sick child". And then a mother says: "Yes, but who would take a feverish child out of bed, just like that? I wouldn't do that either". Another parent then says that fathers can very well take care of sick children and it doesn't harm a child to transport them in a car when they are properly wrapped up. The many voices lead to a dialogue where it started with two monologues. The mirror that the group members are holding to each other is very effective. By observing other parents' battles and their stubborn attitudes, parents will also start seeing themselves. This is confronting, but it also brings about change, because the parents also feel: I do not want to be like that.

There are also always parents who are able to share how they have been busy recognizing the destructive patterns and how often they occur in their lives, and that they remained calm where they used to start a fight. These examples will be singled out and put under a magnifying glass: "What made you react differently now? What did you notice in the other parent? How did you feel, now that things went differently? How did the children react?" Reactions from the group can also reinforce the positive changes. By giving all the couples time to answer these questions, it will become clear that some parents are still caught in the battle, but also that some parents have been able to take actions to free themselves. Nearly always, parents who have been able to put an end to destruction feel strong and good about the change. A mother says: "I can again react from the heart. It has been such a long time since I did that. I want to hold on to that".

In this first hour of the second session, parents always start exchanging experiences and we encourage that. Parents can help each other really well, precisely because they recognize so well where the other is caught. The therapists concentrate on positive remarks and new moves and focus their attention on that. If a parent says that he hasn't had the time to do the assignment, the therapists will say that they regret that and maybe they will find the time to catch up on the assignments in the weeks to come. They add that the parent will probably learn a lot from listening to the other parents. Then, we will again turn our attention to the parents who did find the time to work on the assignments. In this way, we make clear that we focus our attention on parents taking responsibility, but without negatively addressing the more passive parents.

After the feedback of the parents, there is a break.

Break

Chair exercise

After the break, it is time for the theme of the second session:

> *What happens with the children if parents keep fighting?*

This theme is first tackled by means of an experience exercise, in which parents, in the role of a child, experience how it affects them physically, emotionally and cognitively if they are caught between fighting parents.

Goal

Goal of the exercise is to focus the parents' minds on the children again, on what they go through, how it feels for them to be caught between fighting parents and to motivate them to stop the fight and to take another path for the sake of their children.

Instruction

One of the therapists explains that the parents will do an exercise to let them experience how it feels to be a child of divorced and battling parents. In the centre of the room, there are four children's chairs. Four parents will sit down on these chairs (not a parent couple). The other parents form two opposing lines with the "children" on the chairs in between them. We will go through all three destructive patterns and the effect it has on the children. The parents will be battling in three different ways. First, the parents argue openly by shouting accusations at the parents in the other line opposite them. Then, part of the parents will shout accusations at the other line, but these parents will fend off, ignore, look down, look up or stare fixedly, they will sigh or turn around. They will say nothing. In the third round, both lines of parents will form a wall of silence, in between which there will be an icy silence. After about two minutes of silence, parents will start whispering messages in their children's ears. "Because", as a father suggested, "if the parents do not talk with each other, the children will become the messengers".

Before the start of the first round, the therapist asks the parents what kind of things they accuse each other of. The sentences will be written on a flip-chart: "You are always late", "You are only thinking of yourself", "You think your children are yours alone", "It has to be your way all the time", "You are a real borderliner", 'You are a narcissist", "It's about time you start paying", "Why do you always hand back old clothes", and so on. When brainstorming on these sentences, parents often laugh out of recognition. Then, we ask the parents not to act as themselves, but as any parent blaming the other parent. This last instruction is important because parents would otherwise feel inhibited; they think that we would assume that they act like that in real life, and shame keeps them from participating in the exercise. But if we ask them

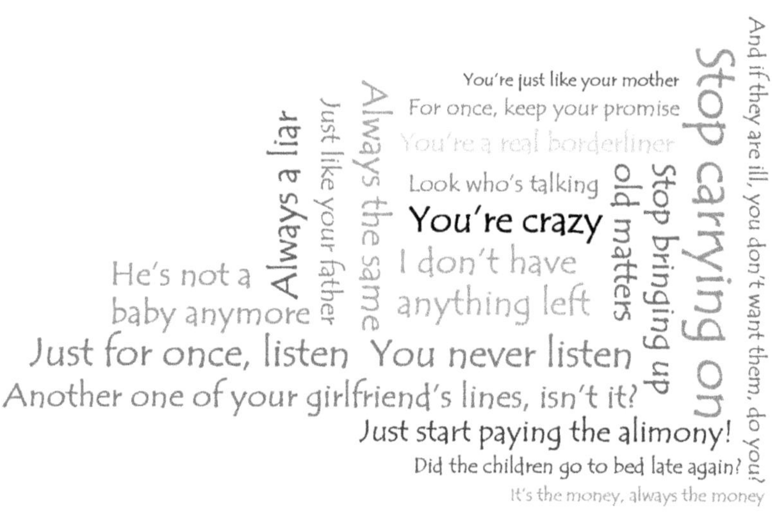

Figure 8.2 Examples of accusations

to play a role, they will do so. After all, it is all about the children and what they feel.

To the parents on the children's chairs, in between the two lines of standing parents, we explain that they are a child, an imaginary child, not their own child. The therapists ask each (parent) child: "What is your name?" The parent thinks of a name. "How old are you? What do you like doing?" After the four parents have imagined a random child, the therapist asks them to put themselves in that child's shoes. They only need to feel like that child and to focus their minds on where in their body they feel like that. In doing so, maybe sentences will cross your mind that match these feelings. The therapists ask the parents to look down or to stare, but not at the standing parents. This is to make sure that they will not look at their ex-partner and be hurt again, and that they are still able to take on the role of the child.

Then, the first round starts. The therapists ask the parents in their role of fighting parent to shout accusations at the other line. Not just to one parent in the other line, but to the entire other line. Partners should not be standing opposite each other, because that would interfere with the "as if" element of the exercise. And it is exactly the "as if" quality that is needed to make parents learn and realize what is going on. Parents can do so in their own language. In one of the groups, parents spoke Moroccan, Spanish, Dutch and Polish at the same time. The sentences that have previously been written on the flip-chart can help the parents find words. After a short while, one to two minutes, the therapist stops the fighting parents and addresses the children.

The therapist kneels over by them, and with a calm voice asks how they feel and where they feel it. The therapist addresses the parents in their child role, using the child's name, and asks: "What do you feel now?" If parents answer with a thought, a reflection, behaviour or an emotion, the therapist asks: "Where do you feel that in your body?" The other therapist makes sure that attention is not distracted by the other group members by jokes, remarks or anything. For many people it is difficult to feel their body and it requires a lot of concentration. One of the therapists asks about the emotions, the other therapist writes the reactions on the flip-chart.

All parents will take on the role of a child in the children's chairs. After round three, all parents will take a seat in the circle again. The empty children's chairs in the centre stay where they are.

Time and again, this exercise proves extremely powerful. It makes parents aware of the effect of their battle on their children. During the exercise, it will become increasingly difficult for parents to participate in the exercise. The parents sitting in the children's chairs are moved by what they experience and find it hard to start fighting with the opposite side after that. Most parents feel shame when doing the exercise. Some parents start to cry spontaneously. Some become numb, some want to walk away, but all parents have strong feelings and matching thoughts.

Finally, there will be a long list of reactions from the parents about what they experienced in the role of a child caught between two fighting parents (see Figure 8.3).

Points of interest

Make sure that all parents take on the role of a child and parent once. For many traumatized people, it is difficult to feel their body. Create a safe atmosphere in which there is no giggling. Correct in a supportive but clear way. Nearly always, there is one parent who has grown up in a

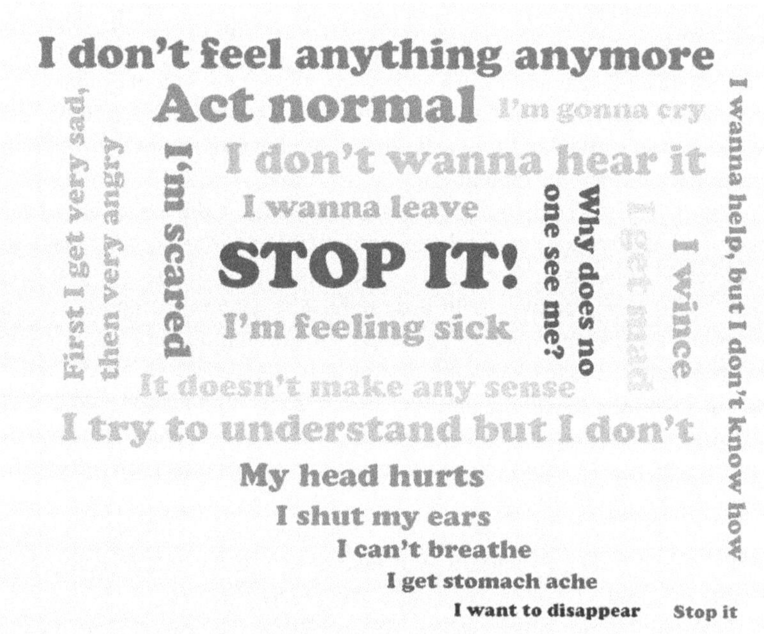

Figure 8.3 Reactions of the "children"

high-conflict divorce or with violence and who ends up reliving events. Explain what is here and now and what the goal of the exercise is.

Get moving

The therapists briefly explain the home assignment for the third session. See *A Workbook for the "No Kids in the Middle" Intervention Programme.*

Closing words

Session 3

Warm-up

Today, the theme in the children's group is:

> *Tensions between parents, loyalty and choosing*

Parents and children are going to draw a weather forecast on each other's backs and then guess what has been drawn.

When explaining the exercise, you can make the link with the position of the children: they often feel they are in the middle and they may feel like they are the messenger. The exercise may, however, also be done without any explanation. Of course, it is also possible to do other exercises that match the theme instead.

The six families stand in one line as a family, one behind the other: a parent at the front, the children in line behind the parent. The last in line is a parent. This makes for six lines next to one another. Explain that the last parent thinks of a simple weather forecast, silently. This parent draws the weather forecast on the back of the child standing before her. This child then draws the weather forecast it has felt on the back of a brother, sister or the other parent before them until the weather forecast has been drawn on the parent standing first in line. Everything in silence, of course. After all the families have finished drawing, ask the parents at the front of the line, one after the other, what the forecast was and ask the parents who started if this is correct.

Variations:

- Drawing figures
- Drawing shapes
- Drawing letters

What has happened since last time?

We start with a short round and ask if anyone has experienced a change for the better. There are always parents who can give an example of a positive change. Other parents are still stuck and find it difficult to get moving. Most attention goes to the positive examples:

- How he had calmly reacted to mail in which she had asked him to just for once be honest in the group.
- How she had decided to give him the children's passports after all to avoid an escalation and, for once, to show her confidence in him.
- How he had sent her mail to explain how badly he wanted to get out of this destructive pattern and that he would do anything to make that happen.

And so on and so on.

We keep singling out and highlighting examples. Then, we ask parents if they have noticed a change in their children and if they react to the reduced tension between the parents. Parents may say that the children are arguing less, that they are more cheerful, or that they haven't complained about a stomach ache or a headache. The therapists can spotlight these positive examples and draw a parallel with children from previous groups and how complaints and concerns decreased in these children, too. There is not much room for examples of parents who are stuck and put the blame for that on the other. The therapist kindly concludes how difficult it is to change and that it sometimes requires some more time.

The fact that this programme helps the children motivates parents to take steps. They don't want to be outdone by other parents who can share examples of positive developments. That is the strength of the group.

Life story for the children

The third session is essentially spent on reading all stories of the parents in the subgroups (see homework session 2 *A Workbook for the "No Kids in the Middle" Intervention Programme*). This exercise proves to be transforming and requires space, in terms of time.

The group will be split. Three parent couples and a therapist go to another room. Until the break and also after the break, therapy will continue in two subgroups, whereby the parents will read the stories they have written for their children out loud. Parents have prepared this at home and, in the group, the other parent couples will help them come to a non-demonizing story in which the other parent remains whole and with which the children can live.

Be sure to strictly divide time between the three parent couples and always start with those parent couples of which both parents have done their homework, since these are the couples that take responsibility for their children. In most of the groups, all parents will have written a story in the form of a letter to their children. The parents who start first choose a buddy who will sit down next to them. The two parents who do not have a role yet take a seat in the children's chairs. They listen with the ears of the child. The buddies are asked to support the parent they sit next to and, at the same time, to understand the other parent. This is very complicated, but important for the children. Then, both parents read their stories to the group.

The parents in the role of a child can show where they feel peace in the story by moving their chairs closer to the parents. When the stories evoke stress, they move away from the parents. In this way, parents reading the story will immediately get feedback on what it does to the children.[2]

One of the parents reads her/her letter. The "children" move closer or away from the parent. Then, the "children" get the opportunity to tell how they felt and why they moved forward or backward. Then, they go back to their initial position and the other parent reads a letter.

After both parents have read their letter, they can briefly confer with their buddy to see if they want to change or add something. The goal is to create a story with which the children can live. There may be different points of view, but there may be no demonizing. If parents haven't written a story, this may create a dilemma if the other parent did write a story. Discuss the dilemma and try to think of a solution together. Sometimes, the group will help find a solution. An option is to let these parents read their letters in the next session.

One parent couple reads their stories before the break. The other parent couples will do so after the break.

Break

After the break, we will continue to work until all the parents have had a chance to read their stories and play the role of a child. Reading the stories will unlock many emotions. Often, parents have been locked in their own truth for years; their own conscious is clear, that of the other isn't. They have shared this story for years on end with anyone willing to listen – relatives, friends, new partners and his/her relatives, school, work and also with the children. This "truth" has gradually become stuck. And now we ask them to let that "truth" go and to write a new, more relational story in which the role of both parents is described and in which attention goes to the children.

Many parents will say that they had a good start. That they fell in love with each other, that they wanted to have children and were glad to have them, and that their relationship broke down later because . . . many variations are possible here:

> "We both worked very hard to provide for you and to take care of grandmother who had fallen ill and which was why there was no time left for us to spend together. This has made us grow apart".
>
> "Because we found out, after a while, that we were too different to be together. Dad likes soccer and action films; mum likes talking and romantic films and a lot more. We started to argue about that more and more".
>
> "When I had to travel abroad a lot, mum felt very much alone and then she started to see neighbour Peter a lot, and as you know, she fell in love with him. That made dad very unhappy, but he didn't say that. Dad became very angry with mum, sometimes too angry".

Some parents use a metaphor or write a poem. Anything is possible. Many parents also explain that their children are not to blame. That they can't help it. That their parents will always love them and that nothing has changed that. It helps when parents are able to acknowledge that it has been very tough for the children and that they feel very bad about that. Many parents end their letter with the wish that things will be better after the programme, so that the children won't suffer so much anymore. The parents in the child position will then move the children's chairs closer and, by doing so, show how nice it is to hear this.

Sometimes, parents are not able to stay out of the demonizing pattern. Like the mother who gave a lecture on the cold childhood of the father, who had not received any love from his parents, which had made him mentally ill and unable to give love himself. That it had ruined their marriage. The parents in the child position will move away. The buddies can help to tell the story in such a way that the father is not blamed for everything and that it becomes more of a relational story.

After all the letters have been read, the group will get together again.

Sometimes, there is some time left for the last information round. Often, however, parents are so full of emotions, that their need to sit together for a while and share things is stronger than the ability to listen and take in information about trauma and the stress system. In that case, we will explain the home assignments and leave it at that.

Information about traumas, conflicts and the stress system

See also *A Workbook for the "No Kids in the Middle" Intervention Programme*, for a comprehensive chapter on escalating and de-escalating.

Interactive group discussion

After sharing the information, we close with an interactive group discussion. The therapists ask all parents if they recognize this and they encourage exchange.

When there is no time left, this may be done in the next session. For instance, following an incident in the group which triggered the parents.

Get moving

See homework for session 4, *A Workbook for the "No Kids in the Middle" Intervention Programme.*

Closing words

Session 4

Warm-up

Today, the theme in the children's group is:

> *Tensions between parents and the reactions of children*

We start the fourth session with the electricity game. Children and parents make one big circle and stand hand in hand. Explain to parents and children that you can pass an electric current by squeezing your neighbour's hand. Secretly, of course. The therapists stand in the circle, both taking their turn. The first therapist closes her eyes. The other therapist points at a child who may start the game. Then, the first therapist opens her eyes and must try to discover where the electric current is being passed. If the therapist guesses right, it's the other therapist's turn.

An alternative exercise is the wave. Explain that in the group we talk a lot about how other people are doing. If you want to know how someone is doing, it is also important to look at that person. That is what we are going to do in the next exercise. We cannot see how someone is doing, but we can see what someone is doing. We also do this exercise because it is important to have fun together, of course. Make a long line across the room, with a few bends in it (like a snake), whereby the parents and children stand in line and the therapists stand in between the families. One of the therapists stands first in line. The therapist does some kind of move and the others in the line copy the move one after the other, creating a wave of the same moves. After that, the first in line goes to the back of the line and the (new) first in line now does a move. Repeat this a number of times.

Possible moves:

- spread the arms wide, then up and back down;
- jump a half-turn and jump back; or
- crouch down and stand up again.

What has happened since last time?

After the warm-up, we ask parents if they have read the workbook and if they have recognized their own triggers, escalations and windows of tolerance. Examples are welcome. Have there been any important developments since last time? We make sure that this round is short and positive, because if we don't we will not have enough time for the rest of the programme.

Presentation of symbols

Next, the parents may explain why they chose the items they brought and which symbolize a compliment about the other parent. The therapists point out that it is very important that the parents try hard to make room for positive stories about the other parent. Positive feelings are not yet required, since you cannot force yourself to have them. It is, however, possible to steer stories and that is a necessary condition for parents to see the other person as a whole person again, with good sides and bad sides. For the children, but also for themselves and for the entire network, it is important that the reduced view of the other person as a kind of demon is broadened again. This also helps to break the demonizing, and it helps to gain confidence in each other again. No one is entirely negative or positive. Most parents in the group are "good enough" and never perfect.

Oran brings a wooden spoon, a notebook and a rubber band. He explains that Ellen prepares good meals for the children, that she always makes lists and thinks of everything, and that she can be flexible when his shifts change. Ellen has brought a ball, a smiley and a cd. She says that she likes to see him playing soccer with their son, that he laughs a lot, and that he likes music and passes his love for music on to the children. Sometimes, parents only bring one or two symbols. The atmosphere in the group is often cheerful and light in this round of compliments. If a parent is still completely stuck and has not been able to think of any examples, other parents can often help because they have gotten to know that parent better, too.

Break

Issues

After the break, we start dealing with issues that individual parents are struggling with – issues that make them get stuck again and again. In sessions 5, 6 and 7, parents will work on these issues, too.

The focus here is on getting parents to move and/or finding new solutions for old problems that continue to cause fights. The group members help each other to get out of the impasses. There are different exercises to deal with the issues in groups. A number of them will be treated in the following, but each team of therapists is free to add new ones.

Inner circle/outer circle

This exercise can be used for issues that may be relevant for all group members. Half of the group forms an inner circle. It is important that the parents do not form a women's group and a men's group. The inner circle discusses a theme, for instance, how to get along with the new partner of your ex. The therapists keep a distance, but try to encourage the parents to share experiences and thoughts. The outer circle listens and is instructed to feel with attention what the discussion evokes in them and which feelings and thoughts come to mind.

After the inner circle has talked about the charged issue for seven minutes or so, parents will switch roles. The outer circle becomes the inner circle and vice versa. Now, the parents who haven't said anything yet will continue talking about the issue, sharing their feelings and reflections. The therapists may add another question, such as: "Do you hope that your child will have a good relationship with the stepparent?" Depending on the intensity, the groups may switch roles several times. Usually, a rich dialogue will develop about the issue, in which different voices are heard and rigid positions are avoided.

Move!

A parent couple brings in an issue which they cannot solve themselves. This exercise is instructive and helpful for the entire group.

Example: a summer holiday problem

He has booked an all-inclusive holiday to Turkey with his new partner and the children and flies back on Saturday. Her holidays with the children start on that same Saturday, and she had counted on her children to sleep at her house on Friday night so that she could leave early on Saturday morning to drive to the campsite in France, where a spot has been booked from Saturday. Her friend and children will join them and they, too, count on leaving on Saturday in the morning. He had booked the holidays earlier, assuming that he could drop the children on Saturday evening. It didn't seem a problem to him and he really can't change it anymore. She thinks that she has accommodated herself so often already and thinks that it is his problem and not hers, because he should just meet his commitments and stick to the schedule. She has no intention to ask her friend, who had also worked around the schedule, to leave later. Votes are equally divided. The children suffer. One daughter has said: "I no longer feel like going on summer holiday".

Exercise

The parents sit side by side, at some distance from each other and slightly facing each other. Both parents can choose a buddy from the group. The buddy takes a seat next to that parent and is instructed to support the parent, but also to help him/her get moving and reach a solution. The buddies put themselves in the position of the parent they support, but they also try to understand the other parent.

Four other parents sit down in the small children's chairs in the middle of the circle. They put themselves in the position of the children of these parents and are instructed to focus their attention on what they feel and think while the parents are talking. When the parents fight and the children feel more stress, they move their chairs away. When the parents are busy trying to reach a solution which also feels good for the children, they will move closer to the parents. In this way, the parents will receive immediate feedback on their way of communicating and their behaviour.

The four other parents are instructed to listen carefully and to feel what they recognize and what resonates with them from their own situation while the other parents are working. What do they recognize and what is different? Do they have something to add from their own experience for these parents?

The therapists ask the two parents who brought the issue up to start. The goal for them is to get moving so that there will be room for the children and to reach a solution together. The therapists don't know what the solution will be, but assume that the parents are able to find a solution together with help from the other group members. Then the parents start.

Mother explains once again why she is really going to leave on Saturday morning and that he should just make sure that the children are dropped off at her place, as agreed. Father says that this is really impossible, because he has booked a package holiday. Booking separate tickets for an earlier return flight is probably not possible and would also cost him thousands of euros. He doesn't have that and she knows that very well. She wards off by saying that he should have thought about that before, that she has often enough accommodated him, including when they were still together, and that she is not going to do that anymore.

When the parents are fighting like that, the "children" move away. The therapist ends the discussion and asks the children to share what they feel: "I no longer feel like going on holiday", "What bullshit", "I want to leave" and "I get angry at both of them". The parents hear the children's voices and can go on. Often, there will already be a softening at this point. Father says that he understands that she finds it inconvenient and that he should indeed have discussed it with her. Mother says she knows it is inconvenient for him, too, but she is not willing to solve the problem for him.

Then, the buddies may talk with the parents, offer support and help them get moving. The four parents sitting behind the children may briefly add something from their own situation. Remarks from parents are often surprising and sometimes even funny. A mother says: "I recognize it; that you consider something irreversible. You say that you do not have a choice, but you could also not go to Turkey", or "We had to deal with the same thing last year, but then I brought the children to the campsite myself. They will be there a day later, but she can still leave early, like she wanted".

With the support of the buddies and the other parents, the parents go into the next round. Often, it helps when the parents can first show they sympathize with the other parent. Father says: "I understand that you are fed up with it. Do you have a suggestion what I could offer in return so you can agree to drive off a day later?" Mother: "I want to think about that. I want to talk it over with my friend, too, but the children must be able to look forward to the summer, so we do have to come with a solution". The "children" move their chairs a little bit closer now.

The therapists ask the "children" to make their voices heard: "It does feel better, but I do not trust it yet. What is going to happen now?", "I can breathe again", "I am tired". The therapists then ask the buddies to play the solution in the role of the two parents. From their position as a buddy, they are often far better able to think of possibilities as they are not caught up themselves in the destructive patterns and negative attributions. They can show understanding for the position of the other parent and help to reduce the tension. They suggest, for instance, that after returning from Turkey, the father drives the children to the campsite of their mother and her friend on Sunday.

The parents will have another round to solve the issue. Sometimes, parents manage to do so. The parents in the prior example reached a compromise; mother would leave a day later, but would get the last weekend of the holidays by way of compensation.

We have found, however, that we must not insist on a solution. Sometimes, parents move, they listen better to each other and there is more mutual understanding. If we would press for a solution, anxiety may increase again and the discussion will become more heated, turning it into a discussion with arguments again. When we sense a positive move and the "children" move closer, we can stop the exercise and say that we are curious to hear how parents will continue from there. "Next time, we would love to hear what you have come up with and how you are going to tell your children".

Then another parent couple may bring up an issue.

This way, a lot of parent couples get a chance to solve their issue. Sometimes all couples do, sometimes a parent couple does not want to. All parents learn simultaneously. The parents who are busy trying to find a feasible solution, the buddies who support but also have to encourage the parents to get moving, the parents in the children's chairs, the parents who reflect on their own situation. All are actively involved with the parents who raised the issue and also with a lot of issues of their own.

The attitude of the therapists is one of being present, firm and supportive. They invite the parents to continue to walk in the field of possibilities. They believe that there is always a possibility. A zen master who attended one of our training sessions said that this is a kind of *Koan*, as we ask the parents to solve a problem deemed unsolvable. A *Koan* is, for instance: "What is the sound of one hand clapping?" These questions help people to go off the beaten track and that is exactly what is needed.

In the group, a large variety of issues are brought up: money, the sale of the house, custody issues. Nearly everything can be a subject of a new dialogue. We help the parents to rephrase the issue into a workable one for which there is a possible solution. We do not accept: "I want to see my children more often", but we do accept: "I would like to pick them up from school on Fridays so that I can keep in touch with the school, too, and spend some more time with the children".

Sometimes, a therapist may, in an open discussion with the other therapist in the group, choose not to have a certain problem dealt with in this way in the group. For instance, the parent who wants to raise the issue of single-parent custody in the group. Or the parent who wants to convince the group that the other parent is lying. When parents are not able to formulate a clear-cut question and remain stuck in: "I am really not going to pay alimony, because if I do, I will not be able to live. You only spend it on the hairdresser and things for yourself, not on the children", then the group cannot help them. But they can if it is about buying a winter coat and how to solve that, because a child does need a winter coat. Therapists and the group can help the parents to rephrase a cumbersome and general issue into a workable one, or they can help to choose another issue.

If things go well, this approach can bring a lot. A mother unexpectedly let her ex miss a large alimony payment. She knew he could not pay it, she had been able to support herself for two years already and realized that the continuing battle, which had already lasted eight years, had brought more misery than anything else. This large gesture of hers also made him take some steps in her direction, and so they found themselves in an upward spiral. This is very encouraging for other parents. A father promised to sell the house after all to get out of financial problems. Parents agreed to no longer fight about the medication of their son, but to leave the decision with the GP.

The therapists let the group members help each other. They provide for a safe structure, but keep from giving any suggestions and making remarks regarding content.

If three couples wish to bring up another issue and there are 45 minutes left, then they each get 15 minutes. Another parent will watch the time.

Get moving

The therapists explain the assignments for session 5. The parents give themselves an assignment and mail it to the therapists. See *A Workbook for the "No Kids in the Middle" Intervention Programme.*

Closing words

Session 5

Warm-up

This is the session in which the children finalize their presentations for the parents. It is important for the children to feel supported by their parents.

Blowing bubbles again. This time, the children try to blow as many bubbles as possible in one blow. Then, the challenge is for the parents is to keep the bubbles in the air for as long as possible by either carefully blowing them up high or by swaying their arms so that the current of air lifts them up. Explain that it is the parents' responsibility to let the children relax (keep the bubbles in the air) as long as possible. In the preliminary talk, you can decide whether you are going to give this explanation (before or after the exercise) or not. Play this game for no more than five minutes. Then, the children go to their own room.

What has happened since last time?

There is a short round to hear how parents have been working on the assignments they gave themselves. Which positive developments have become evident? What do the children notice? Do they manage to see the other parent as a parent who is "good enough"? We continue to ask about the destructive patterns, any escalations and if they could be stopped. If they can tell from their children that the parents are working to change things, and if they have been able to talk about it with people from their network.

We make it clear from the start that room is now needed to apply what has been learned to specific problems. We also ask which parents would like to bring in issues. Time is divided in such a way that all parents who wish to bring up an issue get a chance to do so.

The session goes on as described in session 4 after the break.

Get moving

The therapists explain the assignment for session 6. See *A Workbook for the "No Kids in the Middle" Intervention Programme.*

Session 6

Present when?

We sometimes choose to have both the children and the parents do their presentations in session 6. The children before the break and the parents afterwards. Both the children and the parents are in a vulnerable position, which creates an atmosphere of connection and warmth. Sometimes, we choose to do the children's presentations in session 6 and the parent presentations in session 7. Both before the break. After the break, there is time to talk about the presentations and to discuss other issues. If this option is chosen, parents often incorporate a reaction to their children's presentation in their own presentation. In the following, we describe the option with the children's presentation in session 6 and the parent presentation in session 7.

Start of the session

The parents and the children start in their own group to prepare for the presentations. Parents and therapists discuss how they can best support the children, who will feel vulnerable when they do their presentations, by regulating their emotions (crying, laughing) for the sake of their children. Often, parents know this all too well and it is enough to just briefly point this out. We ask the parents to be there for their children and to help each other keep it safe.

Presentations of the children to the parents

After approximately ten minutes, the parents are invited to the children's room. They are the guests in the children's room, together with the therapists. The children often take good care of the parents. They reserve seats for them and make sure that everyone has a proper place to sit down.

Then, the children will give their presentations (see section 9.2). A couple of times, children made a film with the theme of what happens to you if your parents argue all the time after the divorce. Others presented different works of art: photographs, graffiti or video fragments, music and dance. The children are the guides, taking the parents on a tour around the exhibition and explaining what the works of art represent. Or, the therapists video-recorded the works of art of the children and made a compilation of it for the parents. In one group, there was a film with a script that had been prepared entirely by the children themselves. A pair of twins didn't want to play a part in the film, but had found very appropriate music to match the film. Two older children had interviewed themselves on what the film was about and what the children meant to say with it. After the presentation, there is applause for the children. The children always look very relieved afterwards. It is very exciting for them.

After the presentation, parents and children sit together for a while in their own room for a first reaction. Parents with the parents and children with the children, not mixed up. This is to avoid first reactions which are not appropriate or are too emotional and are expressed during the break. Some parents are very quiet. We have come to understand that they are silent out of emotion and shame. Some parents get very sad. A father started to cry and could hardly stop crying, which made other parents cry, too. Therapists may also be moved and show this. This is often experienced as supportive.

The mirror that the children are holding up to their parents is a very confronting one. It is only after the presentations that some parents become aware of what the divorce battle does to their children. A son who, because of chronic headaches and absence from school, had visited lots of hospitals and had seen many specialists, had made a poster with the text: "It bothers me when you make each other look BAD. It gives me stress and the stress makes me tense and the tension gives me headaches. Because of the headaches, I cannot concentrate and that's why I am not doing well in school".

Other children make photomontages of the battle of their parents and what it does to them – how they become sad, afraid and angry. These emotions were also expressed in several dances by three girls (from different families), aged four, eight and eleven. They had prepared a dance of grief with sad music, a dance of fear with scary music and an angry dance with angry music. Finally, the 11-year-old girl danced a solo, called the "confused dance", in which she expressed how confused she got from the many different stories of her parents.

There was a film about a class that suffered from two teachers taking each other's place in front of the same class, who argued and made the other teacher look bad. Another film was about all the changes taking place after the divorce, what happens if you are new to a class, and how it feels if parents argue on the phone and are not aware that you hear everything. There are lots of other examples of what children have presented. Each time, the therapists are moved and impressed, too.

There are also parents who view it from a distance and say that it wasn't real and that the therapists have obviously thought it all up. Some parents laugh as if it was a funny performance. Other parents are offended by this type of feedback and they correct each other. There is no need for the therapists to add anything to that. Usually, however, there is an atmosphere of connection and warmth.

Break

Reflections and issues

Parents can come back to the presentation session and say what it has done to them. Next, we will ask the parents if they can share any positive changes. We will make time for and zoom in on good examples. Especially what a parent has been able to do differently, enabling another type of interaction, which has made children feel freer. The parents can support each other or sometimes confront each other. By this time, the group will have become freer in reflecting on and reacting to one another. This is usually constructive. The therapists pay special attention to safety, that parents support each other, confront each other, too, but do not damage one another. In this session, there will also be time to deal with a couple of issues as described under session 4. Time will be divided again between parents who want to bring up an issue and who would like to solve the issue with the help of the group, as described under session 5. Sometimes it is a good idea to work in two groups.

Another possibility is speed dating. The parents sit opposite each other in two rows. One issue which everybody recognizes is central. Parents talk for two or three minutes about the issue, then the therapist will give a signal and in one row parents move up one place. Parents then sit opposite another parent and go on to talk about the issue and possible solutions. This is repeated a couple of times and each time parents will be sitting opposite someone else. When there are 12 parents, they may move up to eleven times, but that is usually too often. This exercise nicely reveals multiple voices and may allow for movement.

Get moving

The therapists explain the assignment for session 7 and ask the parents to pay special attention to the presentation they are going to give in the next session. See *A Workbook for the "No Kids in the Middle" Intervention Programme*.

Closing words

Session 7

Start of the session

The parent group starts by arranging the room for the presentations to the children. They can choose to arrange the seats in auditorium style, in a circle or otherwise. It is up to them.

Presentation of the parents to the children

After ten minutes, the children enter the parent room with the child therapists. One after the other, the parents will get the opportunity to show what they have prepared or to say it in words.

A father sang a song with an umbrella over his head: "I'm singing in the rain" and later explained: It is raining now, but we can at least sing and dance again, and that is what I wish for you for the future, too. A mother had made a PowerPoint presentation. Some parents make photo-reportages, a drawing or they write a poem. One parent had tied a couple of mirrors together and asked the other parent and their children to come and sit next to him. He held the mirrors up to them and said that they could all be seen in the mirrors, separately and together. By doing this he wanted to make clear that they all had separate lives, but that they were also connected to one another in some way. A parent couple had made a short film together in which they could often use the word "we". Other parents had not made a work of art, but shared what they wished for their children.

The presentations are all very different, but parents always prove to be very vulnerable and longing for better times. The children usually respond very positively and also emotionally. A sense of connection is very tangible in the room. The therapists provide room and do their best to keep the atmosphere warm and safe. Any criticism is "caught" and bent towards more supportive feedback. If one of the parents uses (misuses) the room to be critical of the other parent, the therapists will stop this and propose this parent listen to the other parents, and perhaps to share later what he/she wishes for his children. So far, this has happened only once. This session involves a lot of connection and emotion. Parents are highly motivated to change and children feel heard. After the presentation of the parents, the children will go back to the children's room and the parents stay in the parent room. We talk for a while about the impact of the presentations.

Break

Issues

After the break, parents can bring up issues again.

Get moving

The therapists explain the assignment for session 8 and ask the parents to complete the evaluation form at home and bring it the next time. See *A Workbook for the "No Kids in the Middle" Intervention Programme.*

Closing words

Session 8

Warm-up

Today, the theme of the children's group is:

> *Tips and goodbye*

The children sit or stand with their parents. The parent couples take turns. They take each other's wrists with crossed arms. In this way, they form a chair for their child. The parents are supposed to carry their child to a certain point (agreed upfront). Explain that the parents can now carry their child. When parents feel too tense to hold each other like that, they can also use a chair or a board for the child to sit on.

If this is not a good exercise for any of the parents and children, the following exercise can be done: make rain.

> In the past seven sessions, we have been working very hard together and made a start to change. You could say that seeds have been planted. Seeds need rain to grow. That is why we are going to make rain now.

For this exercise, parents and children stand in one big circle. One of the therapists, the instructor, stands in the middle of the circle. The therapist says: "We are going to make rain", and then asks everyone to listen carefully. He explains that he will look at the parents and children one by one and then make some kind of sound using his body. The person that is being looked at imitates the instructor and continues to do so until the instructor looks at him or her again. The instructor goes round the circle one or more times, each time in the same direction. A wave of noise will rise around the circle.

Start: silence and concentration

Step 1: The wind rises: the instructor rubs his hands; the others join in one by one.
Step 2: The first raindrops: the instructor snaps his fingers (middle finger/thumb), left hand, right hand, at a steady pace.
Step 3: A real shower of rain: the instructor beats with his hands on his legs, right-left at a slightly faster pace.
Step 4: Storm: the instructor stamps with his feet on the ground at a fast pace.
Step 5: = step 3. The storm becomes a shower again: so, hands on the legs.
Step 6: = step 2. The shower subsides: snapping with fingers.
Step 7: = step 1. The shower stops. It's windy again: rubbing hands.
Step 8: The wind lies down: the instructor lets his arms fall down by his side to indicate that the exercise has ended. The others stop one by one.

If silence has returned, the instructor holds on to it for a while and asks the parents and children if they have heard the shower.

Important developments, looking back and ahead

This is the last session. Before the break, there is time to look into some matters more closely and to hear from everyone about how things are going. Sometimes, there is another round for a parent couple to deal with a certain issue as done before. Then, parents evaluate one another. Each parent will be central, one after the other. Three parents say what they have noticed in terms of changes in this parent, when the parent has done his or her best, what he or she has been busy working on, and what they consider positive. In this way, each parent receives positive feedback from three group members. By doing so, positive changes stay at the forefront. If desired, therapists may zoom in on them, too. The therapists will also ask questions about the future: what can parents do to make sure that the changes are maintained. And questions for the network: do they see changes? In what way can they support the parents to keep going? What do parents and the network see in the children?

If requested or needed, a final network evening will be scheduled.

Break

Evaluation and possible follow-up

After the break, there will be an evaluation per parent couple in the group. First, the therapists point out that the therapy may have its effect in the months ahead.

The therapist will ask each parent couple:

- What positive changes the children may have seen.
- What positive changes the network may have seen.
- How the parent has experienced the project, the therapists and the group.
- What the parent has learned from the group.
- What still may need to be learned.
- If there is still a need for assistance.

It is important to start with the positive evaluations. In each group, there is at least one parent who is not satisfied or who is still stuck. If this person is the first to give feedback, the entire group will be pulled down. If the positive stories are shared first, these stories will also be stored in the memory first. Of course, more critical stories may be heard after that, but these will be seen in a different light: this group works, but not for all, and that is what we said at the beginning, too.

Obviously, we are not in a position to unstick processes between parents which have been dragging on for years in eight sessions. We do see, however, movements in the right direction in nearly all families. Some parents (nearly one-third) are on the right track and are able to stay there. Children of these parents also show the biggest changes and they make most progress. Another group, about one-third, is moving, but still needs support to carry on and to take a few more steps. Then, there is also a group that is moving but also shows some stagnation. There are still many concerns for this group, which calls for a follow-up. But in this group, too, there is usually more room for therapy after the programme.

Evaluation and research

If scientific research is being done, we inform the parents about how things will proceed. We urgently request them to participate in the research, especially if they are not very satisfied, as then we can learn a lot and make improvements.

Now we ask parents to evaluate the programme: What do they appreciate about the programme? What should we stick to? What would they do differently? What did they miss? We always receive valuable feedback, which helps us think about what we could do better in the next group. Remarkably often, parents ask us to be more strict. We find that a tricky request, because they often mean that we should be more strict in stopping the behaviour of the other parent. We stick to presence and compassion. Closing words where everyone can say one last thing.

8.4 Evaluation session per parent couple with people from their network and referrers

For all parents, there is a separate evaluation session with:

- the parents themselves;
- people from the network invited by the parents. Preferably the people who also attended the network evening;
- important referrers, such as a family guardian;
- both parent therapists; and
- one child therapist.

If possible, the final report of the therapy (see section 4.5.3) is sent ahead.

In this session, the child therapist first explains how the child has developed in the group. Together with the parents and the network, we consider if the child needs additional support. We ask the network, too, if they have seen any changes in the children. If children are in custody and/or other types of care are still involved, then it is important to stay in contact with social workers and family guardians.

Then we ask the same questions to the parents. What changes have people around them seen and what changes have they observed themselves? Do they need additional counselling and from whom? Here, we appreciate it when we can directly confer with the referrer.

Some parents want additional counselling, sometimes together with a new partner or another relative. Some parents are now open to trauma therapy or another type of individual treatment. In some cases, additional network meetings will be scheduled.

The therapists take responsibility by suggesting and possibly also finding proper follow-up therapy. Preferably, the therapists provide the (short) follow-up therapy themselves by building on what has already been achieved. They can also involve a therapist they know in this follow-up.

We try to secure the increased activity and responsibility of the parents by adequately briefing other social workers and guardians, and by involving them in what the parents have learned.

We try to convey our confidence in the potential of the parents themselves. If therapists worry about a certain situation, they will mention this in the evaluation and discuss with the parents what is needed. Some parents have put their legal proceedings on hold and have to get back to their lawyers to, for instance, agree on the covenant and parenting plan or the custody arrangement. Hopefully, the lawyers will pick up and support the positive tone. Sometimes, a phone call to the lawyers helps to steer them in that direction.

8.5 Contacts in between and additional network meetings

Parents may grow more anxious and concerned during the treatment. The therapists can often tell this from increased phone and email traffic. To not let anxiety levels rise too high, it is important to be responsive and open for extra attention outside the sessions. This may be the oil that makes the cogs run smoothly again. The entire team is involved in this. Each time, it is decided which therapist will return the call or mail, or have an extra conversation in-person.

Some examples

Bernt, Milan and his mother

The current husband of the mother, Bernt, calls after the third session and says that he will not let her go to the group anymore. She comes home upset after the sessions and they have a young child. He thinks she has taken a turn for the worse, rather than for the better, and she had said all along that she could not be in one room with that man. It is irresponsible, and he will sign her out for the rest of the programme. The therapist says that it is very good of him to call and that she can understand his worries. Obviously, the programme is not supposed to make her worse off and their child is not supposed to suffer from it. She says that she will confer about what they can do about it and that they will be in touch again soon. That same day, the therapist talks with the other therapist of the parent group and with one of the child therapists. The child therapist points out that it would be terrible if son Milan (eight years old) could no longer join if the treatment stopped. He has started to express himself more and more, and he receives a lot of support from a peer in the group. The therapists decide to arrange for a meeting in between sessions with the mother and her current husband, with both the parent therapist and the child therapist. Since everyone is booked up, they are invited for a morning at 8 a.m. that same week. Bernt feels he is being taken seriously, including in the meeting. The mother says that she herself wants to continue, especially now that she knows that Milan is expressing himself well in the group, and she had already heard that he had made friends with someone in the children's group, which does him a lot of good. The therapists predict that there will be more moments that will create tension and make her emotional. Together, they discuss how she can best deal with that and how Bernt can help her with that. She then finishes the programme.

We could give many examples of cases where we follow the principle of being responsive, acknowledging concerns, anxiety and frustrations, and of making every effort to ease tensions and to re-create room for therapy.

Crossing limits

Sometimes, however, parents cross the limits. For instance, when one of the team members is treated rudely. One father demands a lot of attention, but always to point out that the problem lies with his wife. He doesn't want to start working on himself. He is often a disturbing factor in the group, and walks out of the room with his phone to deal with a personal matter. He then sends an email to one of the parent therapists with the text:

> You don't understand a thing. I wait until you say something useful. I have told you so many times before that the real problem is that she is sick. That she is a mental patient. Nobody wants to listen and you do nothing at all. You should rub the shit out of your eyes, you do not see what everyone else sees, including my current wife, my sons, everyone sees it.

We can give hundreds of examples of such emails. We receive emails from nearly all parents in between sessions, often with a copy to other people involved – social workers, guardians, etc. We always take the messages seriously and we divide the work load by alternately making phone calls, writing emails and conducting extra sessions.

Our principle is that if one of the colleagues is attacked, the entire team is attacked. That is why it is a good idea to have the other therapist mail back:

> We have received your email and we understand how desperate you feel. You see just one problem and that is that your ex-wife needs help and needs to change. You don't understand that we do not want that and that makes you angry. And if you are desperate and angry, you will hurt others, and that is not okay. We have talked about it in the group. People who are extremely moved will fight, flee or freeze. You start to fight and by doing so you overstep the mark. It doesn't do you, your sons, their mother and other people around you any good. We think it is a good idea that we meet some time before the next session, together with your current wife. We hope you will be able to come in.

We also set a limit for emails. Parents often want to share screenshots of messages, chapters from books and write long emails. We make clear that we do not have time for that. If parents want to talk to us between sessions, then a short email of no more than six lines will do. In this way, we protect ourselves and make clear that we are not open to opinions and stories about the other parent.

An important additional aspect of the parent group is the interpersonal contact between group members. Sometimes this may reinforce polarization between two parents, as group members turn to each other for support and form a pact with each other outside the sessions. It is best to discuss this in the group and to ask if this contributes to more trust between the parents or not, and to a safer parenting climate for the children.

There are also parents who start to confront, correct and advise others. Sometimes, it helps to advise these parents not to have contact outside the sessions until the treatment is over. Not allowing contact outside sessions does not work. This will end up in fights again. It seems to work well to pass responsibility back to the parent group and the parents in question, with the therapists being clear and transparent about the possible consequences of contact in between sessions.

Network meeting in case of stagnation: three clans become one clan

It is only if the network actively supports the programme that improvement will last. If parents get stuck in negative monologues, we schedule an extra network meeting for the family.

Anna arrives first, with her brother and sister, a niece, three friends, a colleague and her lawyer. Milan arrives with his best friend, three lady friends, a colleague and friend, and his coach. They are received by the two therapists who work with the parents and the two child therapists. The GP, the guardian and the child psychiatrist are also present. A child therapist chairs the meeting. She welcomes everyone, notes the tension in the room and starts with a short meditation to relax. She then asks one of the parent therapists to speak.

The parent therapist refers to the three groups as the mother clan, the father clan and the professional clan, and he summarizes the monologue of each clan.

The mother is afraid that the father has a narcissist personality disorder, that he doesn't create a safe parenting climate for their daughter, offers no structure, gives her unhealthy food, puts her in dangerous situations and thinks too much of himself, which is why he always fails to stick to his word. Examples support her view and her network can confirm this. The mother doesn't understand that we don't see through him, and see that she and her network are telling the truth.

The father thinks that the mother is seeing problems that aren't really there. She is obsessed by structure, bed times and eating rules. She is compulsory to the point of being disturbed and aims at perfection. She puts everyone under pressure. She would like to control each and every one. She is turning her daughter crazy. The father, too, has a lot of examples. Their daughter complains about that and says that she prefers to live with her dad. His network asks us to intervene; if we don't, it will destroy the girl. The No Kids in the Middle team thinks that the battle between the parents is not the issue, and that this hurts and damages their child.

The parent therapist concludes:

> Right now, we can all try to prove ourselves right. If we do, we will have a bad evening and things will get even worse for Ella. Then we are not doing the right thing. I invite everyone tonight to enter into a dialogue, to be receptive to the other stories. Let's first ask the network of the father: what makes him such a nice father? Why is Ella so lucky with this dad? After that, we like to hear the same from the network of the mother.

There will be beautiful, cheerful, warm and moving stories about both parents. The mother's sister stammers: "I am starting to realize that I am always hearing everything from one side only". Others make similar comments. An open exchange follows between the networks of the parents. The therapists hardly get a chance to speak themselves.

The parents and their networks are in control again and embark on a new line. People from the different networks exchange email addresses so that they can stay in touch. A friend of the mother's says: "We have always gone along with one parent and made the other parent look bad. We have to stop that. We'd better make the other parent 'look better'".

In the evaluation, four months later, we hear from the mother that the networks have continued to come together. They coach the parents to stay out of the battle whenever possible. They had asked the mother, for instance, to be available by phone and not to switch her phone off, because it made father anxious. "I always felt cornered and checked on by him, but it is actually not much effort", she said.

Network meetings without parents

In a number of cases we have organized network meetings without the parents being present. This was requested by the networks themselves. They were willing to meet and find out where there was room, but not if the parents would be there, too. That turned out to be a good suggestion. The parents themselves may invite people from their network. For the two networks it is easier to exchange, listen and think of feasible solutions which are good for the child or the children.

These meetings can be scheduled to take place during or after the programme. The structure is similar to that described in the previous example.

First, the father's network explains what makes this man such a good father, with appealing examples. Then, the mother's network will have the opportunity to do the same. The people present may ask questions, such as "Why is he never allowed to call his father and does he have to do that in secret?" or "Why did the mother keep her sick daughter at home on Father's day, but did she take her daughter to her own father after all?" The people involved are full of questions about demonizing stories that have been told for years. While exchanging questions and answers, they often get a broader view and hardly any story turns out to be complete. Then, there may be room to start talking about a feasible parental arrangement which is good for the children.

People in the network are often fed up with the battle, the turmoil it brings and the energy it takes. It wears them out, too. Sometimes also financially. In several network meetings it turned out that grandparents financially supported the legal proceedings, but are fed up with that. That is why they are often more open to compromise than the parents who are stuck in conflict.

For instance, that the father sees his daughter once every two weeks from Thursday to Monday, instead of the short weekend he can now spend with his daughter. For mother this was not open for discussion and father kept on fighting for a 50–50 arrangement. It was decided to opt for the latter arrangement. Here, the network members make sure that the parents accept this plan. A contact person is chosen from each network and communication will go through these contact persons and no longer directly via the parents. They need peace and quiet, too. Of course, not everything goes off smoothly from then on, but we do think that this works better than if a judge imposes it.

This teaming up with the networks is one of the tracks of the No Kids in the Middle programme which we will work out in detail in the future.

Notes

1 van der Elst, E., Wierstra, J., van Lawick, J. & Visser, M., (in press), *Group Therapy for High-Conflict Divorce: A Workbook for the "No Kids in the Middle" Intervention Programme.*

2 Thanks to Jeroen Wierstra and Erik van der Elst for developing the idea of using the children's chairs.

Chapter 9

The children's group

9.1 Goal for the children's group

The focus of the No Kids in the Middle programme is on the therapeutic process in the parent group (see section 8.1).

The goal of the children's group is to enable children to experience and express how their home situation affects them. It will help them understand their own reactions. In the study (Schoemaker et al., 2017), children have shown us that they are fine when they are with one or their parents, but that they suffer in the interspace.

Both the good experiences and the painful ones are dealt with in the group. Children help each other and that builds their resilience. If children can better experience how the situation affects them, they can also better explain to their parents or important others involved what they appreciate and where they suffer. And if parents stop the battle, they can better see and hear their children, and that strengthens their relationship with their parents.

Based on the themes that are at play in the interspace, we make a life story with the children who are open to do so to enable them to deal with the divorce of their parents. We talk about the things that went well, about what has been difficult and how it is to live in two families.

When parents calm down and conflicts decrease and become less destructive, the situation will change. Children will be better able to cope and therapy will become feasible. If children are traumatized, trauma therapy will become feasible, too.

When children are able to tell a coherent life story, they can understand how their behaviour, feelings and thoughts are connected to the behaviour and the reactions of parents, and with the situation they are in (Cohen, Mannarino & Murray, 2011). They feel safer (Oppenheim, 2006). They learn to see that they are not to blame for the conflicts and it is not their duty to make sure that things run smoothly. They can focus more on their own life and activities and they start to see more clearly that they do not need to take sides because both parents have good intentions and that they can have a good time with both of them. And, similarly, that it is okay if there are things they don't like when they are with either one of them.

When things have calmed down enough for the children, we can also ask about the really unpleasant memories and recurring thoughts and feelings about the parental conflicts, possibly also involving other people, like new partners or grandparents. At that point, children may already start dealing with traumatic experiences.

That is not always possible. Sometimes, parents continue to fight during the treatment. That is why it is important to always make room for these differences in the children's group. Some children like to talk a lot and talk in detail about their home situation and their life story. Other children do not want to do that at all. Particularly when the situation is very tense, children often find it hard to talk about.

9.2 The session breakdown

The breakdown of the children's group is as follows:

- warm-up (see section 8.2);
- theme;
- break (see section 8.2);
- presentations; and
- game.

Themes in sessions 1 to 4

The child sessions are structured such that themes are introduced through creative assignments, physical exercises, a game and a group discussion.

Themes of the first four sessions are:

- getting acquainted and the two houses;
- one house with both parents: how did it start?;
- tensions between parents: loyalty and choosing; and
- tensions between parents: reactions of children.

These themes are relevant for all children. Where possible, we work with the entire group so that we can make the best of the group process, the different ages and development levels, as well as the diversity of the stories. We support the themes with different forms of artistic expression, talks, psychomotor and/or creative exercises. The goal is not so much to make sure that everything is being done, but that there are means available to shape the children's process. There is always attention on what suits a certain group, age or child best. Throughout the sessions, the child therapists consider the pros and cons of each option together with the entire team.

Then, the children get to work in small groups, allowing for recognition and acknowledgment, and a form of cooperation that works for all group members. The groups can be composed on the basis of the children's age or their development level, or they may be composed of children who are going to make a presentation together for the parents.

Like the parent group, the programme of the children's group is not a strict recipe either. In each session, there may be ideas to help the group forward so that children feel able to share what they want to share, and to become aware of what they experience, feel and think about the situation they are in. There are also ideas to build their resilience.

THE STORY ABOUT THE DIVORCE

A description of the interspace.
How is life with divorced parents for the child?
How did the family start off? Did the parents end up together?
Did they fall in love? Did they want children? What did they like about each other?

Why did the parents split up? Have they ever lived together?
What tensions are there between parents? Are there arguments?
Has there been any beating? Or was there in the past? Do parents stay silent or do they communicate through the child?
What are the child's nicest or nastiest memories of the family? Of the parents?
Does the child still think about that?
Does it see images, or does it dream about it?
How can the child dissociate themselves from that? What tips can they give other children and what tips can they use from other children?
Who can the child turn to with his or her story?

The order of the themes allows for a life story to be created which revolves around the family – a life story for each child who is receptive to it. How is life in two houses right now? How did the family start off?

How long did the parents live together? When did they get a divorce? Did the parents ever live together? Do parents argue, or are they silent? What does the child think, feel and do when there are tensions between the parents, and what does the child wish for the future?

There is always room for children to say nothing. Some would rather play. Sometimes, when playing, a child may casually start talking about all kinds of things. It helps if the children's room is large enough for children who want to work on their story and children wanting to do something different. The children who work on their story can, for instance, sit at a table and the other children can play, read or watch a film at some distance from the table. It is important that children do not disturb one another. We go into that later in the section titled *Structure and agreements*.

Session 5 and up

Session 5 is exclusively dedicated to the last preparations for the presentations. In sessions 6 and 7, the children and the parents will give their presentations to each other. After the break, the focus will be on supporting the children's resilience. In session 8, the children can give each other tips, finish their life story and say goodbye to each other and the group.

Presentations

In each session, the children will work on the presentations for the parents after the break (see section 9.3.8).

Game

We close nearly each session with an active game that children like to play.

9.3 Points of attention in the children's group

9.3.1 Structure and agreements

The therapists take a semi-directive stand when it comes to the content of the sessions. They have a programme with possible themes for the children, but there is always room to do things differently if that is better for one or more children. There are rules in the group, too. After all, the children that participate in the programme have often been living for a long time in an environment full of conflict, and they respond to that with a lot of emotions and sometimes with restless, aggressive or withdrawn behaviour. The children need boundaries and structure. Some of the rules are different from those in school, and it is important for children to know these rules. In school, they can make mistakes. In therapy, they can make no mistakes. There is no right or wrong. The therapists make sure that the children do not interfere with one another in therapy. There are rules for that and everyone needs to stick to these rules. Children must have consideration for each other, hear each other out, not laugh at each other and not hurt each other. Children may talk, but also hesitate and be silent (Rober, 2012). There is a lot of room for the way children express themselves. They often express what happens to them when parents argue and it often shows that creative expression makes them feel better. They get more air. The children help each other hear their own voices again. They tell what they suffer from and what worries them, but also what goes well and what they enjoy.

What we see is that the children are well able to follow the pace of the parents. When parents work hard, fight less and cooperate better, this is reflected in the children. The children become calmer, and can better describe what they feel and what they wish for. When parents return to escalating fights, children will slide back, too. They no longer have the courage to express themselves like they did before or they decide to take sides with one of the parents again. It often makes them more restless and emotional again, too.

If the children are very restless or indicate that they no longer want to come to the group, we talk about this with the children and the parents. Together with the parent therapists, the child therapists try to figure out what they can do differently so that the children enjoy coming to the children's group again. Or, they can talk with the parents about what the children need and what the parents can do for their children.

The child sessions have a therapeutic effect on the children when parents show progress and the context for the children becomes more peaceful. In the children's group, children feel recognized and recognize each other in themselves.

Some children do not want to talk or dwell on things. They will often say that they do not have a problem. This may be an adequate reaction for older children. They have distanced themselves from their parents' conflicts, they do not feel responsible anymore, and want to go on with their own lives with their friends and the things they value the most. This is different with younger children who seclude themselves. They usually do so out of fear that anything they say will be used in the battle. In these cases, other children may help these children find their own voice again.

Sometimes, children think that their parents argue so much because they are difficult or complicated. After all, parents often say that most of the battle is fought "for the sake of the children". Children do not experience this as such, but they can start to feel guilty about it. By having both younger and older children as part of the same group, a common ground is revealed where children of different ages and development phases can support each other.

It often turns out that a parallel process is going on. In the children's group, for instance, a lot of children are coping with their fear of their parents' anger and in the parent group, discussions are often about bursts of anger by the parents and how it scares them, too – both their own anger and that of the other parent. Or there is a very relaxed and peaceful atmosphere in the children's group, where, at the same time, the parents are busy working in a constructive way. If anxiety levels are high in the children's group, this almost always seems to be a sign that the process in the parent group is charged with fear, too. Even from a distance, children seem to sense that there is tension in the parent group. By marking time and discussing this process with the parents, fear will subside again in both groups. These parallel processes often become apparent in the meetings of the child and parent therapists.

9.3.2 Attitude

The child therapists take a friendly, following and positive attitude. Like the parent therapists, they take a multi-partiality approach. This allows the children to freely express themselves about their parents without feeling judged or condemned. In the children's group, the therapists suggest themes to talk about with the children, but they do not insist. It is the children who determine what they want to say in the group. The therapists follow the process of the children.

An optimistic attitude is needed because, in the meantime, a lot of children have lost faith in a better future. It is then hard to see change and to feel the tension and anxiety subside. The confidence of the therapist and the work that the parents are doing in the parent group can bring hope back for a better future for these children. Yet, it is important to continuously discuss with the children that the parents are sometimes unable to stop fighting. The therapists are very clear about this: children are never to blame for that. Parents, too, are very capable of explaining to their children that they are not to blame for the problems. That may be a theme in the parent group.

Sometimes, children have a very negative attitude towards one of the parents and do not or rarely want to see that parent. As parents in the parent group start moving and stop demonizing each other, the need to take sides will become less significant. This creates room for nuance and the child will be better able to express him/herself in a positive way about the parent that it first rejected. It is conceivable, though, that the child keeps refusing to have contact with one of the parents. In that case, too, it is important that the child does not feel judged for that by the therapists.

The cooperation between the child therapists and between the child and parent therapists is very important. See preliminary and subsequent talks, section 4.5.1.

During the sessions in the children's group, the therapists support each other and can talk to each other about anything, at any time. They confer during the sessions, too. In this way, they show how "parent figures" can cooperate and support each other, even if they don't agree sometimes.

9.3.3 Age differences

Since all children of the six families together make up one group, ages in this group always vary greatly. This has advantages and disadvantages.

An advantage is that the older children can be an example for the younger children. The younger children often provide some distraction with their playfulness. Older children often learn a lot from the explanation the therapists give to the younger children. Younger children can often lean on the behaviour of the older children. In addition, we noticed that it works well to assign special tasks to the older children in the group. It may have a positive effect on their self-image. They help the younger children, explain things and get to understand themselves better in the process, too.

If one of the children differs a lot in age or development level, they will not feel at home in the group. It will think of the others as too childish, feel intimidated or will not be able to follow the group when they are much younger. After conferring with the parent and child, we sometimes choose to offer a separate programme on top of the parent group. We do so if at least one of the parents' children is in the children's group. The child that follows the individual programme does participate in the presentations, though.

For pre-schoolers, a two-hour session is often too long to properly retain attention and the conversations are often too difficult for them. If desired, choose to let the pre-schoolers watch a film before the break in a quiet corner and have them work on the presentations after the break. The pre-schoolers can watch the film in the same room as where the rest of the group is working on the themes. If they want, they can listen to the others now and then, but they don't have to. Always discuss with the parents why you choose to let them watch a film and what film would be appropriate.

The therapists continuously keep an eye on the group dynamics. It helps to ask children about feelings of resistance and a lack of safety. It will reduce the tension in the group and children will feel seen, heard and taken seriously. The therapists also regularly ask the children for help:

> We notice that some children are not happy in the group, or do not want or dare to say what they would like to say. What can we do to make everybody feel at home?

Another option is for the therapists to discuss this together.

> We planned to talk about this subject for a little longer, but I notice that some children are not comfortable with that. Do you feel that too? What could we do to change that? We can go on talking in smaller groups or first ask the children how they feel about it, or do you have other suggestions?

We often work in groups divided by development level, for instance a group of adolescents who like to talk about life and love. They like to combine working on the presentation with chatting and reflecting on themselves and their work. Another example is a group of young children who like to be read to or must do a game now and then to be able to concentrate. The therapists need to be attentive to signs of children indicating that it is time for another activity. The therapists regularly ask for feedback by asking, for instance:

> Are you still okay? It looks like you are getting a little stuck or tired. Am I right?

An important intervention is saying out loud to the other therapist:

> I think they are getting tired. What do you think?

The other therapist can reply by saying:

> I think so, too. We could play a little game, but there is only one more session to go and then the presentations must be ready.

Next, they can ask the children:

> What do you think? How can we solve this?

If the children have different needs, it may be a good idea to split the group:

> Ok, I understand that you prefer to spend some time listening to music and chatting, and that the younger children would like to play a game. Shall we split the group for a while? Then I will go with you to chat and the rest can stay here to play a game.

9.3.4 *Brothers and sisters*

Brothers and sisters often receive support from each other. They are placed in a group where they at least know each other. When there are a lot of brothers and sisters in the group, an only child may feel left out. Sometimes, the safety of a brother or sister prevents a child from blending into the group. On the other hand, the safety of having a brother of sister around may also encourage a child to make contact with other children. They may appreciate it a lot to see each other in the group, outside the custody arrangements, and sometimes for the first time in a long time, without their parents. It may strengthen their ties and motivate them to come to the session.

Brothers and sisters sometimes have a way of dealing with each other which is disturbing for the group. For instance, by playing and teasing each other. Or they may argue a lot. At home, this is sometimes allowed. In the group, however, this causes unrest which doesn't feel healthy or it may provoke even more agitation, which may lead to an un-safe environment. This means that for all brothers and sisters it needs to be determined if they may be in the same subgroups or not. Young adults that had divorced parents in conflict advised us to point out to these children, too, that they could receive a lot of support from each other in the family. So far, we have had good experiences with that.

When brothers and sisters argue a lot, this may also be directly connected with the battle between the parents, for instance, if they each have sided with another parent. They may be afraid that everything they say may reach the parent they no longer see. It helps to talk about this during the intake interview by asking the children how they feel about their brother or sister being in the same group. Since brothers and sisters attend the intake interview together, they may end up talking to each other. In the group, there is a lot of talking about siding with a parent, how often a child sees both of its parents, and how they feel about the contact with their brother(s) and sister(s).

9.3.5 Social media

It is impossible to imagine the lives of today's children without new media. They show their phones to one another, share music and videos, and send Facebook friend requests to one another. It is a way to make contact and to exchange. They often have contact with each other in between sessions. This may be nice and supportive, but some may also be compelling. Children may find it hard to refuse a request or they feel rejected if a request is refused. We talk about this in the group. It is important to point out to the children that everyone is free to give his or her address or number, or to refuse friendship requests, and that everyone can have their own reasons for that. During the sessions, children may sometimes use their phones when they want to retreat for a while. For each child and situation, we decide if this is appropriate.

9.3.6 Wishes for the future

Children often have wishes and ideas for the future with their parents. It is important to point out in the group that there is a difference between wishes and reality. Many children wish for their parents to get back together or to become friends again. Children say, for instance:

> I would like my parents to get together again, but then again, I don't, because they will start arguing again. And I don't think it will happen because my father has a new girlfriend and there is also a new baby.

Wishes rarely come true, but for the development of children it is essential for them to be aware of their own wishes and needs. That is why it is an important topic of conversation. For instance, in the following way:

> If your parents are divorced, it can turn your life upside down. There will be a lot of changes. And as a child, you often don't have much of a say in what is happening. We are curious to know what you would wish for if you could determine what the future would look like. Of course, we cannot make this actually happen for you, but we think it is important to see and hear your ideas. You may choose

> how to do that; you can draw, paint, write a story or a poem, say it or think of something else yourself.

The children often incorporate wishes in their presentations.

9.3.7 General routine of the sessions

At the start of each session, the child therapists prepare the rooms. Then, there is a preliminary talk with the therapists of the parent group. After that, the team of therapists invites the families to the parent room. The children will get to see the parent room and the parents the children's room. After that, parents and children start together in the best suitable room, preferably the parent room. Each session starts with a warm-up with the parents and children together, followed by a group discussion in the children's group about the theme of the warm-up exercise. If they want to, children can share how things have been going since the last session. Has anything nice happened? Or something they didn't like?

When a child says that there is less arguing at home, the therapists give a lot of attention to that. In this way, children can share experiences. What did they notice? How did that go? And how did they feel? Usually, children react spontaneously to each other and the therapist does not really need to intervene. The children encourage and help each other. Sometimes, a therapist must encourage a child a bit more when it wants to say something but cannot find the proper words yet. The trick is to give children room without putting pressure on them. After that, the children start to work on themes of the programme, and after the break they work on their presentations. The children are briefly prepared for the break:

> In a short while, one of the parent therapists will announce the break and you will go to a room where your parents will be, too. You will have a short break and can have a drink and fruit. Some children find this a little bit disturbing, because both of their parents will be there. Do any of you feel like that, too? And who looks forward to it?

There will be a dialogue between the children about the break and how they imagine it will be. They will do an active game together, which will make them feel relaxed before they go into the break. The parents and children will be together for 15 minutes in the family room. The therapists will not be in this room.

After the break, the child therapists invite the children back to the children's room and ask them how they experienced the break:

> Who can share something about the break? How did it feel to be in one room with both of your parents? Who liked it? Who thought it was strange? Who of you felt scared? Was any one of you afraid that their parents would start arguing again? Who of you saw his/her father or mother again after a very long time and how did that make you feel? When a child says that he/she felt scared and wanted to walk away, this will become a theme for a group discussion. The group can think of solutions to make the break bearable, for instance by asking another child to team up with the child during the break or by thinking in advance what he can say to one of the parents or what he will do in the break, and so on. The therapists also ask the child if they may say to the parents that the child finds it difficult to face the break, so that the parents can help. By doing so, the therapists lay the responsibility for reducing the tension on the parents.

During these talks, the children often tell each other what they have seen and heard during the break. There will be children who say: "I saw your parents fill out a form together. . . . And they didn't even argue. . . . Did you see that? The other time, they were still sitting apart, each at one side of the room. . . . I wish that my parents could sit together like that, without arguing". Experience shows that children observe and feel a lot during the break. This is an important source of input for the group discussion and for the creative process when making the presentations. After the discussion, the children continue to work on the presentations. Towards the end of the session, they can again play a game to round off as a group. This will create a lively and open group dynamic, providing room for the group to deal with current issues.

Children may also ask a question of the parents during the sessions. If they have a question, for instance, "Why don't you two just say hello to each other?", then one of the child therapists passes this question on to the parent group. Child therapists may interrupt the parent group at any time to ask a question from a child. After all, children always demand attention when they need it, and parents need to deal with that in normal life, too. The parents respond to the question through the parent therapists or they can write a response to the children.

The therapists stay in close contact with all the children and monitor their attention span. Two hours can be a long time for children to keep their attention. If desired, the therapists introduce one or more extra breaks. Often, children ask for a break themselves. There is room for that, since the atmosphere is open and responsive, where the children's voices are really heard. Sometimes, the children play a little game, like Hangman or Connect4, or they play a game on their phone or tablet, they listen to music, chat with another child or do something else they like.

9.3.8 Goal, backgrounds and examples of presentations

Goal

The group mainly revolves around the presentations that the children are going to make for their parents. The goal is for them to find their own voice, to be able to feel what they feel and to shape the thoughts they have. This may increase their resilience.

Therapeutic impact

Nearly always, the children's presentation has a great and therapeutic impact on the parents, but that should not be the goal. The children are not the therapists of the parents.

Introduction for the children's group

To leave the choice for the presentations with the children, it is important to keep the introduction as open as possible. Giving too many examples may lead to children selecting one of them instead of thinking of something themselves. On the other hand, they do need to know what tools and techniques are available to them, for instance computers, tablets, photos, a beamer, paint, writing material, large sheets of paper and wallpaper, mats to chalk on, music and so on. The examples will excite the children and it will unleash their creative skills.

Means of expression

Children should get plenty of room to express themselves in their own way. Therefore, it is important that they choose a means of expression that suits them and evokes the least possible stress. The means they choose will shape much of sessions 2, 3, 4 and 5. In some groups, children wanted to make a film for the parents. Children who didn't like acting chose the role of the camera man, or they selected the music, so that it truly became a joint project of the group.

In another group, children wanted to work on their own or in pairs. They painted, made graffiti-like posters or wrote a poem. These works of art were then exhibited to the parents. Parents walked past the creations of the children as if it were an exhibition and the children stood next to their work of art, ready to tell something about it or to answer questions. Some children prefer that the therapist explains their creation and they only need to confirm that the therapist explained it well. In another group, three girls of very different ages chose to perform a dance act: a dance of grief, a dance of anger and a "confused" dance. The therapists couldn't have thought of that themselves. A few other children made a sequence of photographic stills. They invented a story and assumed poses to act out the (still) story. The therapists took photos and assembled them, one after the other, creating a very powerful short film.

Music can enhance the images even more. The children can select the music themselves. Of course, the therapists can also come up with examples. Some children like to make a presentation in PowerPoint, in which they can show text, photos, videos and more. This, too, may be backed up by music. In a recent group, two daughters made a lucky tub with assignments for the parents. They had to, for instance, pay each other a compliment on something and share a good memory of the time they were still together.

A wallpaper can be made with the theme of that session. Children can draw and stick things on it, write down birthdays, a message to the network (message of the week), draw a comic strip, interview one another or write down bits of news, ideas or statements of children (anonymously). Each session, something is added on the wallpaper and, if the children want to, it can become part of the presentation for the parents.

The process is the key

It is not the end product, but the process and the road towards the end product, that often proves to be the key. The most beautiful interactions between children happen when they share what they have gone through, or when they brainstorm about the content of their presentation. It is exactly the freedom of choice that gives them the feeling of being in control and makes them enjoy working on the presentation and feel little tension. These factors allow for more room for the children to feel that they can express themselves.

Pressure to achieve quality

Sometimes, therapists feel pressure to make sure that children give a good presentation in session 6. They pass this pressure on to the children.

It is important that children are able to work in an atmosphere where everything is okay as long as the presentation explains at least a little of what the children experience. Good experiences, too, can be incorporated in the presentations.

Safety

Children are often vulnerable when making the presentation. During the process, it is the task of the therapists to make sure that the children do not cross their boundaries. Although we mention a couple of times to the children that the presentations will be shared with the parents, but that the children have control of what they want to show or not, the end result, when shown to the parents, may still take them by surprise. Therefore, we first let the children show the result to one another before they show it to their parents. In this way, they are prepared and are able to tell something about it and sometimes to change one last thing.

No presentation

In exceptional cases, a team can decide that a presentation is not helpful for the child or for the parents. This happens sometimes when a child who doesn't want to see a parent wants to pass on a demonizing message to one of them. If the therapists estimate that the child is not yet able to foresee the impact of it on later life, they may protect the child and choose a form in which the child is still heard without damaging themselves, the other children in the group or the parents. It is recommended that therapists talk these situations over with the entire team. In doing so, a solution will come up in which the therapists can work together, keeping it safe enough for the children and the parents.

At the end

After the presentations, there is often relief and sometimes an elated mood. This is also an indication of how much tension the children feel when they give their presentations to the parents and how hard they have been working on it: "Will they like it?", "Will it make my father sad?", "Will my mother get angry?" We agree with the parents that they will give positive feedback on the presentations of the children. While we often see that children are a little nervous before or during the presentation, they are usually proud and relieved afterwards.

Immediately after the presentation of the children and before the break in session 6, the children and parents sit apart to briefly share how the presentation has made them feel. After the break, the parents give their presentations to the children. Or, parents give their presentations in session 7. After these presentations, too, the children briefly gather in the children's group to talk about what their parents have shown them.

9.4 The sessions

Session 1 – getting acquainted and the two houses

Warm-up

See section 8.2.

Getting better acquainted in the children's group

After the warm-up, the children go to the children's room. We tell them one more time what they have come for.

> Welcome everybody! In the coming months, you will come to this place with your parents every other week. You have all met us once before, but we are going to introduce ourselves one more time. My name is Daniella, and this is Jerry. As you can see, there is a camera standing over there. It records everything we say and do. That is to make sure that we don't forget anything. Sometimes we want to watch the video again to make sure that we have understood everything properly. We can learn from that. The video recordings are only used by us. We do not show them to your parents or other people. Today is the first time you see each other, so please say your name, how you like to spend your time, and if you have a brother or sister in the group.

And we ask who is nervous about meeting each other for the first time, or about being in one room with all parents and children. The therapists also raise their hands after each question and one of them explains that being in a new group always makes him/her nervous.

> I am always a bit tense at the start of a new group. I am curious about all the children. Some of them I have already met once, but not all

> of them. And I am curious as to how they will be together. I am a bit nervous about the moment when parents and children come together in one room, because I know that some of the parents have not been in one room with the other parent and the children for years, or that some parents quickly start arguing with each other, and some parents don't look at each other. Those are the things that I am a little tense about in a new group.

If communication in the group runs smoothly, the therapists may talk a little while about this with the children. If there is too much tension, the therapists will propose to get better acquainted with each other first. Then, we do the name exercise again. The therapists do a round of introductions. They say their names, tell where they work, and that they often work with children of divorced parents and that they love doing that. Then, the children introduce themselves to the group by saying their name and age, and by sharing how they like to spend their time. Everyone receives a sticker on which they can write their own name and stick it on their clothes so that the others can memorize the names. The introduction is continued in the form of a game whereby one of the therapists stands with his back to the children and closes his ears and eyes. The other therapists point at one or two children who will then go to the corridor. Then, the first therapist may turn round and start guessing who has/have left the room. The therapist thinks out loud, and mentions the names of the children who are still in the room so that children will hear the names several times. Repeat this and let all children have their turn, unless they do not want or dare to. Children like to go to the corridor with someone else. There are many other types of introductory games (see Appendix 4). Therapists can decide for themselves which game they choose. Then, the children sit down in a circle and the therapist will explain:

> We are here together because each of you has a father and a mother who do not live together and who often argue, or blame each other for everything under the sun, or they argue or do not speak to each other anymore. They know that it is not good for you. They do want to stop it, but they don't know how. That is why they attend the programme.

Some children will say, "My parents do not argue. They don't say anything to each other" or they say, "They don't argue, they don't yell, but they often disagree". Other children say, "My parents really argue. They say nasty things to each other and sometimes mum or dad has to cry".

> What do you call this? The arguing, the whole thing? Or do you have another word for it? What shall we call it here? In this group, you can share what bothers you and also what goes fine. You may talk about it and give each other tips, but you don't have to. But you will all make something to show to your parents how it makes you feel when they argue or disagree a lot. Your parents are here to learn how you can suffer less from their arguing and tensions, and also how they can work better together so that things will be better and nicer for you at home. Sometimes, we see that parents manage to do that and that there is much less or no arguing anymore after the programme. Sometimes, they are friendlier to each other or they interfere less in each other's lives. We also see that parents sometimes do not manage to make things better. If that is the case, the therapists of the parent group and the parents will try to find another solution.

The children have a group discussion about this theme. They can do so by answering the following questions:

> What do you think about this? Who of you ever wonders if the arguing and the tensions will ever stop? Some parents also say nasty things about each other or they send each other nasty messages. Who of you has ever experienced that?

It is important to de-blame children and to lay the responsibility for the arguing on the parents:

> Who of you ever thinks that the arguing is his/her fault? We think that the children are never to blame for the arguing between parents. They have to make sure that it stops. What do you think?
>
> We think that parents may disagree with each other about the children or about the rules or about parenting, but we also think that parents are responsible for the way they argue or solve their conflicts, and that they should not bother the children with that. How do you feel about that?

By answering these questions, children may come to realize and maybe also express that they are not the cause of the fights. Children can help each other on this point, too. The older children especially can help the young children understand that they are not to blame, that they used to think that sometimes too, but that it is not true. Another question may be:

> Who of you has ever tried to help the parents or to stop the arguing? Some children try to do that sometimes, but it often doesn't help and then children may feel guilty about that. We think that parents must stop the arguing themselves. Children do not have to solve it for them, and that is why your parents are in the group. Because they are going to help each other to stop the arguing. What do you think of that?

Again, we encourage the children to talk about this, but without pressure. Some children will give examples and like to share. Others are still quiet, but react nonverbally to what is said. Some don't react at all. If there is a lot of unrest in the group, we do a game before moving on.

Break

There is a break when the parent therapists knock on the door. The parent therapists decide when it is time for a break and the children's group follows. By leaving the parent therapists in charge, the children never need to wait in the corridor until the parents are ready. They continue to work in their own room.

Two houses and the interspace

Tell the children that they have talked about living in two houses during the intake interview. Explain that in this session we will again talk, draw and write about living in two houses, or living with one parent and not seeing the other parent. The goal of this theme is for children to recognize things in each other when it comes to living with two parents who live apart and are very tense when they are together, and to find recognition for that. All questions asked are about topics which children have told us are important. That doesn't mean that all questions need to be asked and answered. We do not mean to badger them with a barrage of questions. The questions serve as a guideline for the therapists, though, to make sure that big topics aren't overlooked.

Start a group discussion using the questions about the *interspace* (see Chapter 6) if the children are open to talk about this.

The game "Cross the line" is often a good warm-up (see also Appendix 4). Mark a line on the floor using a rope. The entire group is on one side of the line. For each question, say: "Cross the line if". For instance, "if your parents are divorced". All children who can confirm this cross the line. Children who do not, may, for instance, say that their parents were never married and that is why they don't cross the line. You may keep on asking a child questions, but you don't have to. It is a good way to share experiences about living with divorced parents in a way that evokes little stress. Children do not need to say anything, just cross the line or not.

Children who find it difficult to join the game can play something else and will get something out of the exercise just by being in the same room.

Questions

The questions from Chapter 6 can be used to get the group discussion going. The questions are meant as a mnemonic for the therapists. They are not meant to be asked one after the other. Some children share more while they are playing, between the lines. Others only say something when they are specifically being asked a question. Therapists adjust to the children, the group and each other. It is important for the therapists to confer on this.

A wallpaper can be made surrounding the theme of the day. Children can draw and stick things on it, write down birthdays or other bits of news, a message to the network (message of the week) or other ideas. Statements of children (anonymously) can also be written on the wallpaper and questions they have for their parents (anonymously). Children may, if they want to, incorporate the wallpapers into the presentations to the parents.

Body-oriented exercise

Stand up with the children. Tell the children that attending a group or talking about difficult topics like the divorce may create some tension in their body. Ask who feels tension in his/her body sometimes and give an example from your own experience: "When I find something difficult to do, or exciting, then I feel it in my belly – a little itch." Ask the children to lay a hand on the place where they feel or can feel tension.

Show the children what move helps you to be less tense. And ask the children what they do when they are tense and what helps. Think of examples like breathing out properly (like when blowing bubbles), standing firm with two feet on the ground, and standing on your toes first and then on your heels, counting to ten, thinking of something nice for a while, jumping around and so on.

Session 2 – one house with both parents, "how did it start?"

Warm-up

See section 8.3.2.

Do you remember the names?

Do an exercise to memorize the names again.

One house: "how did it start?"

The theme of this session, and part of the divorce story of the children, is the question of how their parents got to know each other. For children, it is important that they are wanted, that their parents were very excited when they were born, and that their parents did have a nice time together, however short or long that was. The session is about getting a conversation going between the children, where they are curious about each other's and their own history. Start the conversation, for instance, by saying:

> All parents once started off together. Some parents have lived together and with the children for years. Some parents fell in love with each other, but they didn't get to live together. At least all the parents got children together. And you are these children! Do you happen to know what your parents liked about each other? And how they got to know each other? Or are there still things they like about each other? And do you have nice memories of the time that you lived together as a family? Or did nice things?

Ask the children if they have questions for their parents and if they can or dare ask them. Maybe there are other people in their network who can answer these questions. After the group discussion, the children may write something, make a drawing, or cut pictures from magazines and stick them on a sheet about that first period. Sometimes, brothers or sisters like to do this together, sometimes they don't. Therapists can help children write something down. At home, children may look for photos to add.

Break

Explanation of the presentations

Explain the goal of the presentation in the sixth session.

> We will not yet start to work on it today, but it may help if you know what each other's hobbies are, what you like doing or what you are good at so that we can figure out how we can use those skills when you are going to make the presentations. Maybe, when you know more about each other, you will decide that you would like to give the presentation with someone else so you do not have to do it alone. You can work together. Children often do that here.

Game: yes, no?

This game serves as a warm-up for the presentations. The goal is to let the children think about different forms of artistic expression and subjects for the presentations.

Take three sheets of thick paper and write on the words "yes", "no", and "?" on them. Lay the sheets of paper at three different places in the room. The children stand in a corner of the room and answer closed questions asked by the therapists by walking to the relevant sheet of paper. At first, the questions may be fairly general to get to know each other a little better. Based on the answers of the questions, short follow-up questions may be asked.

Example questions:

- Who likes to play computer games?
- Who likes Brussels sprouts?
- Who has a dog?
- Who finds it hard to concentrate in school?
- Who likes pancakes?
- Who has a favourite animal? (ask what animal)
- Who sometimes argues with his/her father and mother?
- Who is in primary school?
- Who feels sad sometimes because things don't go well between mum and dad?

- Who feels angry sometimes because things don't go well between mum and dad?
- Who has a favourite sport? (ask what sport)
- Who likes taking pictures/dancing/singing/acting?
- Who has ever made a vlog?
- Who has ever tried to stop the arguing between their parents?
- Do your parents call each other names or hurt each other by beating or kicking?
- Who has ever interviewed someone?
- Who has ever made a newspaper?
- ....

Let the children also ask a question themselves.

Make sure that the follow-up questions are open questions. Often, therapists tend to ask: "Who dares to tell something about the fights?" Usually, children answer this question with: "No". It works better to ask: "We asked you who has ever witnessed a fight between his or her parents, and you were standing at the 'Yes'. Tell me, what is it like when your parents fight?" And then, ask another child who is standing at the "Yes", "And how is that with your parents?" "And you are standing at the question mark. Tell me, what do you mean by that?"

Choosing the type of presentation

Let the children think about how they wish to make the presentation. For some children, this will be difficult. See if groups are being formed already. Find out if there are children who like to draw, to take pictures, or to craft or the like. If children find it hard to think of something, it may be helpful if you talk with them about how they feel about the divorce or the tensions they feel.

For younger children, it may be helpful to first make some drawings of the four basic emotions (sadness, happiness, anger and fear) and then to figure out with them what they feel when their parents argue or do not talk with each other, or say something unpleasant about the other parent. Or when parents are cheerful together.

Make things as concrete as possible for the child based on what you have learned about how things are going between their parents. Then, you can start to figure out together how the child wants to express this. Try to find something appropriate, something the child likes doing or appears to be good at. Some children like to show what they think their parents are doing well. Many parents and children can learn from that. For instance, a proper transfer where parents are nice to each other and wish each other a nice weekend.

Session 3 – tensions between parents: loyalty and choosing

Warm-up

See section 8.3.3.

Tensions between parents: loyalty and choosing

In the children's group, we start a conversation by asking the children who passes on messages between parents sometimes. Ask the children how they feel about that. The goal is to make children become aware of what they are doing, whether they want to do it or not, if they can refuse or not, and that, regardless, it is NOT their task.

Tensions between parents

Parents are different. Talk with the children about their father and their mother. In what ways are they alike (they both love their children) and in what ways are they different? Explain that the differences between their parents can also be reflected in the different rules they impose. Make a list of what makes it difficult for the children. Are there differences in rules? The following additional questions may be asked: Do you have to get used to being at dad's house or not? Do you regret having to leave dad again or not? Do you feel sorry for yourself or for your dad? Do you think a lot of mum when you are at dad's house, or do you have to think of dad when you are at mum's house?

> You are here in this group because your parents find it hard to talk to each other. They hardly speak to one another; they don't say hello to each other or they often argue. Some fathers and mothers send each other lots of emails or WhatsApp messages, others don't at all. Sometimes they pass messages to each other via you. They will say, for instance: "Just tell your dad that . . ." Or your dad says something similar and you are supposed to pass that on to your mother. How does that work in your situation?

Let the children ask each other questions if they feel the need to and encourage them to talk in the group.

> What do you know about the divorce? Who told you that your mum and dad were going to get a divorce? And why did they get a divorce? Do they tell the same story? And for the children whose parents never lived together, do you know why dad and mum are so angry with each other, or why they find it so difficult to be parents for you together?

Loyalty

All children in the group have problems with loyalty. The therapists can tackle this theme by having a group discussion. They explain things and ask who of the children recognizes problems with loyalty, how they feel about that and how they are coping with it. There will be room to express emotions related to the battle between parents, and for talking about positive and negative sides of both parents. They can also recognize feelings in each other and support each other. The therapists decide upfront if the conversation will be held with the entire group or in subgroups, and if they will have a group discussion or opt for another, more creative form of expression, like the wallpaper mentioned before. A few example texts follow. The goal is for the children to be able to express themselves by talking, playing or drawing. Although the therapists decide on the topic, they will follow the children in the subgroups. The children may talk, hesitate and remain silent, or draw.

> It is often difficult for children when parents argue or don't talk with each other anymore. We have learned a lot about that from children in previous groups. Ten-year-old Tom said that he always felt caught between his parents. Who of you has ever felt like that, too?
>
> We have just started the session together with the parents again. Children in other groups told us that they sometimes find it hard to choose whom they were going to sit with. Has anyone of you felt like that sometimes? And some children have found a way to deal with that. They sit, for instance, with their dad first and with their mum next, or they wait until their brother or sister has chosen first and then they choose themselves. Who of you has ever done that? And are there children who do not know what they want themselves? Or do not dare to do or say what they want? For instance, because they are afraid to hurt their dad or mum?

Nadia preferred not to visit her father so often anymore and Jonathan would rather not visit his mother anymore. Who feels like that, too? Do you think that Nadia and Jonathan don't love both of their parents?

We sometimes hear that it is difficult to enjoy being at mum's and at dad's if they make each other look bad all the time. Do you agree with that? How is that in your situation?

Who of you finds it difficult to say something about his father to his mother, or the other way around? This happens a lot because fathers and mothers may react in anger or sadness. Because of all this business between your parents, you may have all kinds of different feelings, which may be confusing. Does anyone of you feel like that sometimes?

Ella and Sadir said that they often feel lonely because they think their father or mother do not really understand how they feel or are too involved in their divorce and too little with them. Can you imagine that?

And some children only feel anger. They are angry at both parents, their father or their mother, or themselves. Some children feel sad because of the rows, or they miss their father or mother very much when they are at the other parent's house. And some children are just happy that there is less fighting at home, or that they do not have to see their father or mother so often anymore. You can have all kinds of feelings at the same time. That makes it even more complicated!

These feelings are very normal if your parents argue a lot and make the other one look bad.

Using these questions, start a group conversation, make a wallpaper or choose another form of expression that suits the children and the group. Ask the children how it makes them feel and what they consider when making choices. Ask the children if they recognize things in each other and invite them to react to one another.

Choosing

Then, ask the children if there are any other situations where they feel like they have to choose. If the children cannot think of anything, you may say: "Who is right when they argue? Who is to blame for the divorce? Who do you want to be with on Christmas Day?" Here, you can show videos or clips, for instance of Villa Pinedo. It can help them to express themselves.

Children often say they wait and see where their brothers or sisters are going to sit during the warm-up with the parents and that they divide attention between their parents. That if one of them chooses to sit with the father, the other will sit with the mother. Continue to ask questions, for instance, how children without siblings solve this. Or families with an uneven number of children. Some children divide their attention between their father and mother by time, so if they sat with their mother in session 1, they will sit with their father in session 2.

It is important that, at the end, the therapists stress that it is quite a lot to consider, that it is very sweet of the children to care so much for their parents, and that they don't want to hurt them, but that it makes it pretty hard to still feel what they want themselves. Ask the children if they can still feel inside what they want themselves, and if they have the courage to say that.

Also talk about the feelings they may have when they have to choose one parent, when in certain situations they prefer to be with both of them, but they know that it doesn't work or that they know that one of the parents doesn't like that. For instance, to come watch a performance at school or a sports game. Do children recognize this? How do they deal with that? Do they dare to make a choice or do they not show anything? How do they make a choice? From there, you can make the step towards having the children express these feelings.

Working on the presentation

After the break, everyone continues to work on their presentations. The therapists walk around to see who needs help and join in.

Session 4 – tensions between parents and reactions of children

Warm-up

See section 8.3.4.

Tensions between parents -2-

It is the responsibility of the parents whether and how they argue. Together with the children, list the topics which the parents often disagree on. For instance, hang cards in the room with the following topics: money, the children, clothes, the weekend, Mother's and Father's Day, holidays, school, birthdays, Christmas, Sugar Feast and a card with another topic on it. The children stand, for instance, in the middle of the room and the therapists ask: "Whose parents sometimes argue about money?" The children whose parents sometimes argue about money can go stand near that card. Or, the therapists ask: "What causes the most tension between your parents?: Or, "What topic do you hate most when your parents argue about that or do not talk about it? What topic is easy for your parents to agree on?" Each time, continue to ask questions to each child:

> What is that like? How does that make you feel? What do you think? What do you do? How would you like it to be, and can you tell your parents? What can you do yourself when they argue and you are there, too?

Explain that many arguments are about the children, even if the parents live together, because parents always want the best for their children. So, if they do not agree with each other, they will try very hard to convince the other.

Most of the time, both parents are a little bit right, but sometimes only one parent is really right, or one parent is all wrong. Many children like to know who is right, but they can't really figure it out. There are also children who do not mind at all who is right. They don't want to be bothered by it. Arguments aren't bad, people don't always agree, but how parents solve their conflicts is their responsibility. Children should have no part in that. Hand out the open letter of Villa Pinedo to the children, "To all children of divorced parents" with the theme "it is not your responsibility".

It is important, though, to learn how to argue or to disagree in a good way. And to make up afterwards. Children often feel that parents don't agree and that there are tensions between the parents. Sometimes, they also witness their parents arguing and it bothers them. Sometimes, parents try very hard not to argue in front of the children, but then the children can still sense that they have had an argument. "Who has ever experienced this? And how do you notice?"

Body-oriented exercise

What does anger or tension between your parents look like?

We are going to do an exercise about how parents show that there are tensions or that they are having an argument. The children think about what they see in their parents. The therapists act it out by striking poses.

One of the therapists thinks of how it would have to look like, strikes a certain pose, looks in a certain way and then gives instructions to the other therapist about how he or she should stand and look. Both therapists then strike their pose. Then, someone can take a picture (a student or a child). Then, ask the children who would like to do the same. The child may come forward and chooses another child to do the exercise with. After they have struck their pose, a picture can be taken again. The other children will be asked what they recognize in the pose. Ask the children what they feel when there is tension or an argument between parents. Let them act out the feeling. Children can also act and later film a "good argument" and a "bad argument". Children can use the video in the presentations. With the pictures, the therapists or the children can show the parents the work they have done. Of course, all the children need to give their approval for that.

When the therapists see that the same kind of poses are struck over and over again, they can show other examples (think, for instance, of examples from the theory about destructive patterns). Talk with the children about arguing, having different opinions and about tensions between parents. Or, choose another form of expression to tackle these topics. What impact does it have on children? What is a good way and what is a bad way of arguing or dealing with tensions? Talk about it, for instance in the following way:

> You have just struck all kinds of poses of people having an argument or having tensions. Some things you don't approve of. For instance, when parents call each other names, when they threaten each other, or beat or kick each other. In fact, when they hurt each other on purpose. Arguing in itself is not bad. Everyone argues from time to time because they are very mad at someone or because the other person is very angry. Think about how this is with your friends, or when you are angry with your father or mother. When you have a row, it is not only about "being angry and arguing in a good way", but it is also important to make up again and to be able to say "sorry" if you actually know that the other person is right or if you unintentionally hurt the other person in your anger. Arguments or silences create a lot of stress if they don't solve anything if the arguments don't stop and the differences don't go away, or if you witness the arguments but you do not have a say in it. Or, if they ask your opinion and you have no idea. Or if it is about you,

> but they don't ask your opinion. One person thinks this, the other thinks that, and they keep on repeating it, or nothing is said at all anymore. It often bothers children.

Ask the children what happens to them when there are tensions or arguments between their parents. What do they feel, what do they think and what do they do? Do they walk away, are they going to stand in between? Do they interfere in the argument or rather draw the attention of their parents?

Dealing with trauma

Some children have experienced very unpleasant arguments, sometimes involving others, too, for instance stepparents or grandparents. When parents calm down, have less fights and see their children better, there is sometimes room to start dealing with trauma. If that is the case, you can ask about the most unpleasant experiences: What is the most unpleasant thing the children have experienced between their parents? That may be the worst row, or the nastiest thing one parent has said about the other, or something the children have read in an email of the parents. Is there something they still think about a lot? Or something they see in their mind's eye when they lie in bed? Who feels very lonely or alone sometimes? Who cries in bed sometimes, or somewhere else? And who can they turn to?

Alternative option to talk with children about parental tensions and arguments

Watch a (YouTube) video, for instance a television programme for children about high-conflict divorces. Ask the children to react to the video and write the reactions on a flip-chart in text balloons. The children may use the flip-chart in their presentations, or it may be shown to the parents by the therapists to illustrate what the children have been doing in the children's group. Of course, the children need to give their approval first. See previous example.

Going through the presentations

Go through all of the presentations to make sure that children have a chance to make changes in session 5. Some children want to make changes after all, and by taking time to go through the presentations now, there is room to do so. Watch carefully what a child has created and what text and pictures have been used. Parents, too, need to be addressed with respect in the presentations by the children. The therapists make sure that this is the case. If not, talk about it with the child and explain, then decide together how the presentation can be changed.

Session 5 – finalizing presentations

Warm-up

See section 8.3.5.

Presentations

Before the break, the presentations are finished. After the break, we will have a last rehearsal. By doing this, the children can have a final look at their own presentation and other children may also see how the presentations have turned out.

Session 6 – presentations of the children for the parents

This time, parents and children do not start together, but go straight to their own room.

Preparing the children for their presentation to the parents

We explain one more time to the children in what way the presentations will be shown to the parents. We also talk about the order of the presentations. We make sure that there are enough seats in the room. Children may decide for themselves if they want to sit with their parents or not. Then, the parents are invited to the children's room.

Presentations to parents

The children give their presentations to the parents. The child therapists coach this. After all the presentations have been given, we ask the parents to go back to their own room again.

Follow-up discussion about the presentations to parents

We will have a follow-up discussion with the children and ask them if they have seen how the parents felt about it and how they reacted. We often see that by this time, children are running out of energy or that they become restless as it has been very exciting for them. It may be a good idea to do a game together so that the children can release some of their energy.

After the break, there is room for the children to do what they like. Sometimes, the release after the presentation is so strong that the children become rowdy. Therefore, it is recommended to prepare something, for instance a film or a nice activity. The therapists watch over the structure and make sure that everyone is safe. In between, the children can come back to the presentations, the reactions of the parents or other themes.

Session 7 – presentations of the parents for the children

Parents and children start in their own room, like in session 6.

Preparing the children for the presentation of the parents to the children

We explain to the children that the entire children's group will go to the parent room in a moment, since all fathers and mothers have made something for their children or are going to tell their children something. The child therapists do not know what the parents are going to present or say, but they do make sure that they know when a parent has called off or has announced that he or she is not going to give a presentation. They can say this to the child in question before the start of the presentations in the children's group. Explain to the children that it is an important moment for all parents and children, and that everyone deserves to be listened to and children should not talk at the same time as the parents. Then, the children go to the parent group.

Presentation by parents

In turns, the parents give their presentations to the children. See section 8.3.7. After the presentations of the parents, the children go back to the children's group for a while and the parents stay in the parent group. There will be room to talk about the presentations. Then, there is a break.

Talking about the parent presentations and the letter to the network

Parent presentations

We give time and attention to each child. What do they remember about the presentation of their parents? Have they understood the message their father and mother wanted to convey? Due to the high tension, the children may not have been able to properly listen to what their parents said. Sometimes, parent stories are difficult to understand. Then, the other children can be asked what they have understood from the story. Carefully watch for non-verbal signals and involve the group to highlight multiple aspects of the presentations of the parents. Sometimes, children are so used to interpreting their parent's behaviour as negative that it may be helpful to ask other children whether they interpreted the presentation in the same way. There will always be children who are able to highlight the positive side of a presentation or to recognize the love expressed through it. Watch carefully how brothers and sisters react together. Can they help each other in any way in explaining what their parents have said?

Letter to the network

After giving proper time and attention to all children, there is room for a letter to the network. A letter to the granddads, grandmas, stepparents and other important people. What do the children want to ask them or say to them? The letter from Villa Pinedo may serve as inspiration. The children may, for instance, write a message or interview each other. Anything is possible. If children are too tense or too tired, there is, of course, room to play and relax.

Session 8

Warm-up

See section 8.3.8.

Tips for the future

Talk with the children about what they can do if the parental arguments or tensions continue, or if one parent says something negative about the other parent, or if someone from the network does so. And let each of them give a tip. Go around the circle until no new tips are given. Tips can be written down by the therapists or by the children themselves. Children may also craft a box to keep their tips in. Extra support is needed for children who feel that nothing has changed at all.

Evaluation

Evaluate the children's group with the children and ask the following questions:

> You have attended eight sessions of No Kids in the Middle. You were in a group with other children, and nearly all of the sessions started off with the parents. You have talked, drawn and played about where you live and about the custody arrangements, about the way your parents have contact with each other, about the fact that you feel that you have to choose, and about what you would like to be different. You have made presentations for your parents. You have seen the presentations your parents made for you. We want to ask you some questions about all that. What did you find difficult in the group? What did you like a lot about the group? What will you remember of what has happened or what you have learned in the group? What did you find stupid? What shouldn't we do in the group anymore? Do you have any suggestions for a following group? Have you noticed changes in your parents? Have things changed in your life? How does that make you feel?

Goodbye

Arrange for some big, nice cards or create them yourself from coloured cardboard. Write a name of a child on each card so that there is one card for everyone. Let the children and the therapists write down something nice on each card for the child in question. At the end of the session, each child takes his/her own card home. Optionally, the card may be given during the evaluation. Explain to the children how the evaluation with the family will be like and when it will take place.

Epilogue

This book is a work in progress. Ever since the first group, we have felt that we are engaged in a very useful project and also that there is still room for improvement. Sometimes we are thrilled about what we have achieved in a session; sometimes we are at a dead loss of what to do.

As the book goes into its third edition, new adjustments to the programme are already on the way. Each time, we evaluate with the parents and the children. We are in constant dialogue with each other and other providers. We conduct scientific research, both nationally and internationally. In doing so, we are always open to change. Accordingly, the programme is subject to constant change, maybe even forever. This means that it will never be a fixed protocol. Each time, we make changes that fit that particular group of parents and children. And after an evaluation, new changes are implemented, following the useful suggestions of parents.

Important changes are announced and communicated via our website www.kinderenuitdeknel.nl. In each new edition, we will explain the changes that have been implemented. We hope that therapists working with No Kids in the Middle will adopt the key principles of the methodology, but also feel free to make useful adjustments.

No Kids in the Middle is not a magic potion that will de-escalate all quarrelsome divorces and release all children from being caught in the middle. The results, however, are so positive that we continue to dedicate ourselves to these children and their parents.

Appendices

Appendix 1

Registration form

Dear Madam/Sir,

Thank you for your interest in the No Kids in the Middle programme for the . . . . region.

The municipality where the child(ren) is/are registered determines whether the programme is paid for; it usually is. If your child is *not* registered in the . . . . region, you will find a list of providers in your region on our website http://kinderenuitdeknel.nl/contact. For information, please contact the relevant provider.

To sign up for the No Kids in the Middle programme, follow these steps:

1 To start the registration process, we need you to provide us with the following details:

- Your address and postal code
- Your date of birth
- Your telephone number
- Your referrer and name of the referring body
- Name(s) of the child(ren)
- Date(s) of birth of the child(ren)
- Place where the child(ren) live(s)
- Name of ex-partner

2 If **both parents have signed up separately with their details**, you will receive a date for an **exploratory talk with one of the therapists of No Kids in the Middle**. We prefer to have this talk with both parents.

3 If, after this exploratory talk, both parents decide that they wish to join the programme and sign up one or more of their minor children

for the children's group, they will receive: a registration form and a questionnaire, to be completed and returned together with a copy of the child's ID card and a referral letter for No Kids in the Middle from the GP or a youth and family centre in the name of the children. This may differ per municipality.

4 We need to receive the questionnaires from both parents. After **we have received the documents, we will put you on the waiting list**.
5 As soon as the next group is started, parent couples on the waiting list are invited to the intake interview.
6 If, three months after the first registration, the other parent has not signed up, your details will be removed from our records and the registration will be cancelled as part of the General Data Protection Regulation. We will notify you about this.
7 We are not allowed to provide information about the registration of the other parent. We advise you to contact the other parent or the referrer for more information.
8 Your forms will be passed on to the therapists in charge of the invitation for the intake interview. Your information will be treated as confidential.

If you have questions, please contact . . . . (or send an e-mail to . . . .)

With kind regards,

Coordinator of No Kids in the Middle

. . . . (name)

Appendix 2

Open questions No Kids in the Middle

Name(s) of the child(ren) taking part in the programme:

Who has parental authority over the children?

When did you get a divorce/did the relationship end?

How long were you together?

Is there a parental plan?

What are the current arrangements concerning parental access? When are the children with whom?

Is there any other social care (including, for instance, custody placement)? If so, which types?

Are there any legal proceedings going on (which may be stopped for the duration of the programme)?

What is the current family composition (names and ages, (half) brothers/sisters, new partner)?

What is your motivation for joining the programme?

What complaints do(es) your child(ren) currently suffer from?

How is the relationship between your child and his/her parents, any (half/step)brothers/sisters and any new partners?

What school does your child attend and how does your child do in school?

What hobbies/sports/other extracurricular activities does your child have/do?

Has your child experienced any development problems (for instance, with regard to their motor system, eating behaviour, sleeping behaviour, speaking/linguistic development)?

Has your child experienced any traumatic events, outside the divorce, and if so, which and when?

Describe some positive character traits of your child. What are you proud of?

Can you briefly tell something about the conflicts with the other parent which bother you?

Is there anything else you think we should know?

Thank you for completing this questionnaire!

Appendix 3

Invitation for participation after intake interview

Place, date

Dear parent,

Soon, you will be attending the *No Kids in the Middle* programme, together with your child(ren).

The sessions will take place on day, from a.m. to p.m. at:

(name institution)
(address)
in (place).

It is important that both you and the children attend all sessions.

Dates of the sessions:

Session 1
Session 2
Session 3
Session 4
Session 5
Session 6
Session 7
Session 8

The information evening will be on (date) from p.m. to p.m. at the same location. You will need to come to this meeting with people from your network (at least two, no more than five) who feel involved with you and your children. These may, for instance, be relatives, friends or current partners. In this meeting, we will give information about the programme. The evening also serves as the kick-off of the programme.

We would like to know in advance how many people we may expect to come to the meeting. Could you therefore please indicate with how many people are going to attend the meeting with you?

We hope for a fruitful cooperation,

See you on (date)!

With kind regards,

& (therapists parent group)

& (therapists children's group)

Appendix 4

Exercises and games

Exercises and games for the children's group or the warm-up

What follows a list of examples of exercises and games that can be done during the group sessions – exercises that encourage parents and children to get better acquainted or to strengthen the group cohesion and games to relax. The therapists can incorporate these activities as they see fit, but they may also think of exercises themselves. The exercises can be done during the warm-up or in the children's group.

Getting better acquainted

Interviews

The children interview each other in pairs, after which they introduce each other in the group (or in two subgroups) to the rest of the group and tell what they have learned about the other.

Collage

The children make a collage or a drawing about themselves to introduce themselves to the group and tell something about themselves.

Cross the line

A line is drawn with a rope, blocks, chalk or the like. On one side of the line is a therapist or a child reading a statement. The other children stand on the other side of the line and cross the line if the statement applies to them. If the game is used as an introductory game, it is important not to touch on subjects that are emotionally charged. Examples may be: Cross the line if you are an only child/play soccer/like pancakes. This game can be played again later with statements that do touch on the battle between the parents or other more personal topics.

Yes/no?

This is a variation of "Cross the line". The room is divided into three corners: the yes, no and ? corners. Then, questions will be asked which the children answer by running to the relevant corner. Example questions are: Do you like horse-riding, do you have brothers or sisters, do you like Brussels sprouts? And if the group has started to feel more familiar: Do you sometimes suffer from headaches? Are you bothered by the arguments between your parents? And so on.

Calming down

Landing exercise

This exercise is meant to let the children step back from the day-to-day rush. The children sit down in the circle or at a comfortable place somewhere in the room. They close their eyes and the therapist starts a short guided imagination:

> *"You wake up on a beautiful island. You lay on the beach and feel the heat of the sand on your back. The sun is shining and you feel the sunbeams on your face. You sit up and look around you. What do you see? The sea, or trees or maybe something else . . . What do you smell? . . . What do you hear? . . . You start walking and you walk around the island. You walk and you walk and you feel that your feet are getting tired. You start to slow down and you feel that your breathing eases. Then suddenly, you see someone approach from the distance. It or he or she is coming closer to you. Do you recognize what or who it is?"*

And so on.

Complete the exercise by asking the children to open their eyes again, slowly sit up straight, stretch, and then go sit in the circle again. Sometimes, you ask who or what the children came across on the island, what they saw, smelled or heard. Sometimes, you don't talk after the exercise.

Who is it?

One child is blindfolded and must guess who is standing in front of her/him by feeling the other child's head. The other children are told to be quiet as a mouse during this exercise.

As quiet as possible

The children get assignments which they have to do as quietly as possible. The children next in line must also be very quiet so that they can hear if the assignments are carried out without a sound:

- walk somewhere;
- pick something up and put it down again;
- stand up and sit down again;
- stand on the chair;
- open the door and close it again;
- open the cabinet and close it again.

And so on.

Feel more free in the group

Rock, paper, scissors

With this exercise, children can start to feel freer in the group and with the other children. Children walk around without touching each other. When they run into someone else, they say in sync: "Rock, paper, scissors". As they say these words, they tap one closed hand against the palm of the other hand. On the word "scissors", both players reveal the object they chose. To play "rock", they ball their hand up into a fist. To play "paper", they extend their hand palm down with the fingers outstretched. To play "scissors", they use two fingers to mimic the shape of an open pair of scissors. There are two possibilities:

- The children throw the same object. It's a tie and the children simply play again until there is a clear winner.
- The children throw different objects. In that case, rock "crushes" scissors but is "covered" by paper. Paper "covers" rock but is "cut" by scissors, and scissors is "crushed" by rock but "cuts" paper. The player who plays the stronger of the two objects is the winner.

The losing players sit down. The winners walk on until they run into another child and they play the game again.

Avalanche of rhythm

The children sit in the circle and the therapist explains what an avalanche is. The therapist starts to clap in a certain rhythm. After three claps, the child next to the therapist joins in. After three more claps, the next child joins in, and so on, until the entire circle claps in the same rhythm. Then, the avalanche slows down again. Each time, after two counts, another child stops clapping, following the circle until it is silent again.

I pack my suitcase . . .

The objects are acted out in pantomime instead of being mentioned.

Exercises about emotions

Goal of these exercises is to talk about, recognize and understand different emotions. The exercise can be done to prepare for a talk about feelings, but also as an introduction before working on the presentations. It is determined in advance if the exercise is done with the group as a whole or in subgroups. There are various options.

Active game

The children walk around the room. The therapist mentions an emotion which the children then act out in their pose, their way of walking and facial expression.

The emotion bus

Create a small bus using chairs. One of the therapists will sit on the bus like a driver. Make sure to wear a nice hat. One child gets on the bus. That child has a certain emotion, for instance happy, scared, sad, angry or in love. All other passengers, beginning with the bus driver, copy the emotion of the child who last got on the bus. Then, another child gets on the bus with another emotion. Everyone on the bus copies this emotion. And so on. When the bus is full, the child who stepped on the bus first has to leave. All passengers copy the emotion of each child as they leave the bus until the bus is empty again. Do not forget to take off your hat.

Hints

The children each receive a card with a certain emotion on it or they can think of one themselves. The therapist can make a list of emotions in advance for the children to choose from. The children take turns acting out a feeling. The one who guesses correctly goes next.

Emotions and music

The therapist plays a short tune after which the children think of an emotion that matches the tune. Or, they act out that emotion.

Collages

The children look for pictures and texts in magazines that represent certain emotions and they stick them on a large sheet of paper. This may also be done in pairs.

Play with emotions

The children separate into small groups. These may be mixed groups, with children of all ages. They make up a play with different emotions and then they perform the play for each other. At the end, the others guess what emotions they saw acted out during the play.

Games of trust

Trusting blindly

The children work in pairs. One child closes its eyes while the other guides this child around the room.

Soft doll

The children form a small, closed circle of about seven children. One child stands in the middle and closes their eyes. This child falls forward and is caught by the other children in the circle. The child tries to be a soft doll and falls in every direction. Trust is key in this game.

Knot

Make a circle and give each other a hand. One child goes into the corridor. The circle ties itself into a knot: walk towards each other, step over each other's arms, curl yourself around someone else, and so on. The children don't let go of each other's hands. The child in the corridor comes back, and they are tasked with untangling the group, without the hands letting off! At the end, the group will be standing in the circle again like they did at the start. This is a game of trust because the children will be standing close to one another and they have to hold on to each other for the duration of the game.

Exercise in loyalty

Determine in advance if the exercise is done with the group as a whole or in subgroups. There are various options:

Acting out loyalty

Choose a way to act out how it must feel for children to get caught between their parents or to disagree with a parent. You may paint, draw, write a story or a poem, or make photographs of stills. This is often a first step towards the presentations and the results may also be used in the presentations.

Appendix 5

Final report

[Place],

This is the final report about participation in the No Kids in the Middle intervention programme by:

Parents:	Children:	
Ms/Mr Name	Name	, born
Ms/Mr Name	Name	, born
	Name	, born

have been referred with his/her/their parents to No Kids in the Middle.

They took part in the intervention in [place], with therapists of the Lorentzhuis and the Children's Trauma Centre of Kenter Jeugdhulp. The programme took place from to . The goal of No Kids in the Middle is for children to experience less stress in their lives as a result of fewer conflicts between their divorced parents. The programme is conducted in two parallel groups, a parent and a children's group, which meet eight times, once every two weeks. The focus of the programme is on the therapeutic process in the parent group. When parents calm down and conflicts decrease in number and become less destructive, the situation will change. Children will be able to cope better and therapy becomes feasible. The children's group is supportive and, where possible, therapeutic, and is always aimed at boosting the children's strength. If the situation is safe enough for the children, they can create a story about their family and the divorce, and deal with what has happened.

Main points of this treatment are:

In the parent group:

1 *Children and parenting are central.*
2 *Empathizing with children* and sympathizing with what they experience as children of fighting parents.
3 *Breaking through destructive battle spirals* and working on other, more constructive ways of dealing with differences and conflicts.
4 *Focussing on own behaviour*: what can I do as a parent to improve the situation for the children?
5 Recognizing one's own vulnerability and *triggers of fierce emotions* and being able to better regulate emotions so that conflict escalation will occur less often.
6 *Letting go and accepting* parallel parenting and trusting that the other parent is good enough. Accepting that you cannot change the other and that it is best to focus on your own life and your own relationship with the child.
7 Transforming the demonizing story about the divorce, where the storyteller is the victim and the other is the perpetrator, into *a story the children can live with.* In this story, good memories are cherished, nobody is blamed and everyone plays a part.
8 *Forgiveness and reconciliation*: because children need it and because long-lasting anger, stress and frustrations are unhealthy.
9 Living with *multiple truths*: from black-and-white to colour.
10 Involving the *social network* (grandparents, new partners, relatives, friends, school, social workers) in the changes and having them support new behaviour.

In the children's group:

1 Children support each other as *fellow sufferers.*
2 Teaching children to recognize what they *experience as children of battling parents* and to put this into words.
3 Relevant themes for children are tackled: the *tensions between* the parents surrounding the transfer, birthdays and holidays, money, loyalties and grandparents, and other relatives.
4 Increasing *resilience* in children.
5 Who can children turn to if parents are not available (*social network*)?
6 The children make a *presentation for the parents*, alone or in groups, in which they show what they experience as children of battling

parents. This can be done in the form of text, a drawing, dance, video or a game, music, theatre and so on.

7 Children who feel safe, and who want to create *a life story* – a story about how the family started off, what went well and what went wrong, and how that made the children feel.

Course and result of the treatment:

Conclusion and recommendations:

The team of No Kids in the Middle:

Parent group	name and function name and function
Children's group	name and function name and function

We went over the report with the children in the children's group. Both parents have read the report. Both parents have been given the opportunity to react to the report. Any reactions can be found in the appendices to this report.

Appendix 6

Final report example 1

Haarlem, 10 February 2019

This is the final report of No Kids in the Middle.

Parents:	Children:
Ms Mary Brown	Emily Johnson, 6 March 2009
Mr Ben Johnson	

Emily and her parents were referred to the intervention programme by . . . . They took part in the intervention in Haarlem, with therapists of the Children's Trauma Centre of Kenter Jeugdhulp and the Lorentzhuis. The programme took place from September 2018 to February 2019. The goal of No Kids in the Middle is for children to experience less stress in their lives as a result of fewer conflicts between their divorced parents. The programme is conducted in two parallel groups, a parent and a children's group, which meet eight times, once every two weeks. The focus of the programme is on the therapeutic process in the parent group. When parents calm down and conflicts decrease in number and become less destructive, the situation will change. Children will be able to cope better and therapy becomes feasible. The children's group is supportive and, where possible, therapeutic, and is always aimed at boosting the children's strength. If the situation is safe enough for the children, they can create a story about their family and the divorce, and deal with what has happened.

Main points of this treatment are:

In the parent group:

1 *Children and parenting are central.*

2 *Empathizing with children* and sympathizing with what they experience as children of fighting parents.
3 *Breaking through destructive battle spirals* and working on other, more constructive ways of dealing with differences and conflicts.
4 *Focussing on own behaviour*: what can I do as a parent to improve the situation for the children?
5 Recognizing one's own vulnerability and *triggers of fierce emotions* and being able to better regulate emotions so that conflict escalation will occur less often.
6 *Letting go and accepting* parallel parenting and trusting that the other parent is good enough. Accepting that you cannot change the other and that it is best to focus on your own life and your own relationship with the child.
7 Transforming the demonizing story about the divorce, where the storyteller is the victim and the other is the perpetrator, into *a story the children can live with*. In this story, good memories are cherished, nobody is blamed and everyone plays a part.
8 *Forgiveness and reconciliation*: because children need it and because long-lasting anger, stress and frustrations are unhealthy.
9 Living with *multiple truths*: from black-and-white to colour.
10 Involving the *social network* (grandparents, new partners, relatives, friends, school, social workers) in the changes and having them support new behaviour.

In the children's group:

1 Children support each other as *fellow sufferers*.
2 Teaching children to recognize what they *experience as children of battling parents* and to put this into words.
3 Relevant themes for children are tackled: the *tensions between* the parents surrounding the transfer, birthdays and holidays, money, loyalties and grandparents, and other relatives.
4 Increasing *resilience* in children.
5 Who can children turn to if parents are not available (*social network*)?
6 The children make a *presentation for the parents*, alone or in groups, in which they show what they experience as children of battling parents. This can be done in the form of text, a drawing, dance, video or a game, music, theatre and so on.
7 Children who feel safe, and who want to create *a life story* – a story about how the family started off, what went well and what went wrong, and how that made the children feel.

Course and result of the treatment:

Emily was motivated and actively took part in the group. She missed out on one session when she was ill. She enjoyed being with the other children in the group, especially with two girls her age. She worked with these girls on the presentation for her parents. Emily has been able to express herself through talking, drawing and playing about important themes during the treatment. Emily told us that she liked the group so much because there were no children of divorced parents in her class, which is why she finds it hard to talk about it in class and she felt ashamed. Others in the group encouraged her to talk about it in class and then there appeared to be more children with divorced parents in her class after all. The themes in the children's group raised questions in Emily's mind about the divorce story and she has asked her parents a lot of questions. Parents have learned to stop the negative verbal communication with and about each other. Especially in front of Emily, they speak less negatively about each other. They have become more aware of their own vulnerability and the triggers of fierce emotions. As a result, they are better able to stay calm when talking about Emily. They both started to answer Emily's questions about the divorce story in a way that she understands.

Conclusion and recommendations:

By participating in the No Kids in the Middle intervention, Emily can now talk about the divorce with her parents. The programme has revealed the issues that both Emily and her parents are still struggling with. Emily can ask support from her parents, and the parents ask for more support from their new partners. The parents have made a good start in explaining the divorce to Emily. When answering Emily's questions, both parents still find it difficult not to blame the other parent. Emily has told the children's therapists, however, that she feels that both of her parents are doing their best for her. In the final meeting we advised the parents to regularly ask people in their network how the communication goes, so that Emily does not find herself in a loyalty conflict again. Both parents were present at the final meeting and want to keep paying attention to this. The parents indicated that they have no need for a follow-up programme. The file will therefore be closed. Emily has indicated that she has a need for a buddy at Villa Pinedo. We agreed that she will take the initiative for that herself and ask her parents for help, if needed.

We hope we have provided you with sufficient information. If you have any further questions, please contact No Kids in the Middle.

With kind regards,

The team of No Kids in the Middle:

Parent group	Justine van Lawick, clinical psychologist/system therapist Margreet Visser, clinical psychologist/senior researcher
Children's group	Elisabeth van der Heide, Healthcare psychologist/system therapist Jeroen Wierstra, drama therapist/system therapist

We went over the report with the children. Both parents have read the report. Both parents have been given the opportunity to react to the report. Any reactions can be found in the appendices to this report.

Appendix 7

Final report example 2

Amsterdam, 10 February 2019

This is the final report of No Kids in the Middle.

Parents:	Children:
Ms Caroll Easley	Oliver Harris
Mr Michael Harris	Charlotte Harris
	Jacob Harris

Charlotte, Oliver, Jacob and their parents were referred to the intervention programme of No Kids in the Middle.

They took part in the intervention in Amsterdam, with therapists of the Children's Trauma Centre of Kenter Jeugdhulp and the Lorentzhuis. The programme took place from September 2018 to February 2019.

The goal of No Kids in the Middle is for children to experience less stress in their lives as a result of fewer conflicts between their divorced parents. The programme is conducted in two parallel groups, a parent and a children's group, which meet eight times, once every two weeks. The focus of the programme is on the therapeutic process in the parent group. When parents calm down and conflicts decrease in number and become less destructive, the situation will change. Children will be able to cope better and therapy becomes feasible. The children's group is supportive and, where possible, therapeutic, and is always aimed at boosting the children's strength. If the situation is safe enough for the children, they can create a story about their family and the divorce, and deal with what has happened.

Main points of this treatment are:

In the parent group:

1. *Children and parenting are central.*
2. *Empathizing with children* and sympathizing with what they experience as children of fighting parents.
3. *Breaking through destructive battle spirals* and working on other, more constructive ways of dealing with differences and conflicts.
4. *Focussing on own behaviour*: what can I do as a parent to improve the situation for the children?
5. Recognizing one's own vulnerability and *triggers of fierce emotions* and being able to better regulate emotions so that conflict escalation will occur less often.
6. *Letting go and accepting* parallel parenting and trusting that the other parent is good enough. Accepting that you cannot change the other and that it is best to focus on your own life and your own relationship with the child.
7. Transforming the demonizing story about the divorce, where the storyteller is the victim and the other is the perpetrator, into *a story the children can live with.* In this story, good memories are cherished, nobody is blamed and everyone plays a part.
8. *Forgiveness and reconciliation*: because children need it and because long-lasting anger, stress and frustrations are unhealthy.
9. Living with *multiple truths*: from black-and-white to colour.
10. Involving the *social network* (grandparents, new partners, relatives, friends, school, social workers) in the changes and having them support new behaviour.

In the children's group:

1. Children support each other as *fellow sufferers*.
2. Teaching children to recognize what they *experience as children of battling parents* and to put this into words.
3. Relevant themes for children are tackled: the *tensions between* the parents surrounding the transfer, birthdays and holidays, money, loyalties and grandparents, and other relatives.
4. Increasing *resilience* in children.

5 Who can children turn to if parents are not available (*social network*)?
6 The children make a *presentation for the parents*, alone or in groups, in which they show what they experience as children of battling parents. This can be done in the form of text, a drawing, dance, video or a game, music, theatre and so on.
7 Children who feel safe, and who want to, create *a life story* – a story about how the family started off, what went well and what went wrong, and how that made the children feel.

Course and result of the treatment:

Oliver, Charlotte and Jacob have actively taken part in the children's group. We will give some brief feedback per item.

Fellow sufferers. All three children found a lot of support in the group. Oliver worked with other children on the presentation. Charlotte and Jacob were always together.

Experiences and tensions. The children looked tense, which manifested itself in boisterous behaviour (in particular in Charlotte and Jacob) and a lot of quarrelling among themselves. They could be properly corrected, though. They listened carefully to what other children said, asked questions and talked about their own experiences, too. The conversations had a calming effect on Oliver. Charlotte and Jacob joined in as well, but were also restless and were constantly moving. They took part in the conversations about differences and about arguments between the parents. Oliver was a little reserved at the start, but listened well to the others. Later on, he was able to properly tell what bothers him about the arguments. Charlotte and Jacob have, in particular, been able to draw about their experiences.

Resilience. Taking part in a group with fellow-sufferers increases resilience in children. They experience that they are not the only ones in such a complex situation. Doing playful exercises with the parents also gives them resilience and courage. This is particularly true for Oliver, and to a lesser degree for the younger children. We noticed that it was helpful for Oliver to hear that he is not responsible for the well-being of his parents. This message did not really come across to the younger children, but that is quite difficult for this age anyway.

Presentation. The children did their very best to make a presentation for their parents. When they gave the presentation, all three of them were visibly tense. The situation in which the parents gave their presentation was also very tense for the children. All three of the children were less tense at the end of the programme and were arguing less among themselves in the group. They also told us that they were arguing less at home and that they are pleased with that. The children haven't created a life story yet because there are still too many questions about the divorce.

Parents have both actively taken part in the group. In what follows, we will give some brief feedback per item.

Making children and parenting central. It is clear that both parents love their children very much and that the love is mutual. Fights and breaking agreements have compromised the trust and cooperation between them. Father finds it difficult to organize his life properly. Mother has come to understand that it is not because he is unwilling. In the course of the programme, there has been more openness and communication, and the parents have been able to communicate about the care for the children again. Although frail, we could feel more relief.

Empathizing with children. The children could be very emotional now and then. Both parents were able to properly support and comfort the children. They gained increasing insight into the impact of their suspicious behaviour on the children. We have the impression that there is more openness and exchange between the parents and the children. Mother is able to talk nicely and calmly with the children. Father is more the comforting and hugging type.

Breaking through destructive battle spirals. Parents have made considerable steps in breaking the destructive patterns. They have become a little more generous towards each other. However, they are both also on their guard and alert. It may easily go wrong again.

Focussing on own behaviour. Parents have come to understand that the tensions will not ease when they continue to try to change the other. They have each focussed on their own behaviour and what they can change themselves to improve the situation of the children.

Recognizing triggers of fierce emotions. Parents seem to be more aware of what triggers them in the other and how they react to that.

Letting go. Parents have come to understand the importance of "letting go" and are busy taking steps in that direction.

Story which the children can live with. Parents have worked hard on a story about the divorce which the children can live with. This is something they can continue to work on.

Forgiveness and reconciliation is still a lot to ask, but may be possible in the future. The parents won't be friends again, but they don't need to be.

Parents realize that there are *multiple truths*. In situations where there is a lot of stress, they sometimes lose sight of that.

Social network. Both networks play a role in the tensions and also in the support. Parents realize that contact with both families is important for the children. Tensions in the father's family complicate this.

Conclusion and recommendations:

Parents have managed to better deal with the tense situation surrounding various issues. In the last group session, both parents were able to say that the other person is good enough as a parent and that they will reconcile themselves to the different parenting styles. They will continue to dedicate themselves to this. Both parents want follow-up talks to consolidate the results. Their new partners are happy to help them. Looking ahead, there is much hope for further change, provided parents are able to sustain and continue the movement they have made in the last few months.

The team of No kids in the Middle:

Parent group	Erik van der Elst, drama therapist/system therapist Flora van Grinsven, clinical psychologist/system therapist
Children's group	Wendy de Visser, remedial educationalist Danielle Steggink, remedial educationalist/psychomotor therapist

We went over the report with the children. Both parents have read the report. Both parents have been given the opportunity to react to the report. Any reactions can be found in the appendices to this report.

References

Adriaanse, M.A., Gollwitzer, P.M., De Ridder, D.T., De Wit, J.B. & Kroese, F.M. (2011). Breaking habits with implementation intentions: A test of underlying processes. *Personality and Social Psychology Bulletin*, 37, 502–513.

Alisic, E., Zalta, A.K., Van Wesel, F., Larsen, S.E., Hafstad, G.S., Hassanpour, K. & Smid, G.E. (2014). Rates of post-traumatic stress disorder in trauma-exposed children and adolescents: Meta-analysis. *British Journal of Psychiatry*, 204(5), 335–340.

Alon, H. & Omer, H. (2005). *The Psychology of Demonization: Promoting Acceptance and Reducing Conflict*. London: Routledge.

Amato, P.R. (2001). Children of divorce in the 1990s: An update of the Amato and Keith (1991) meta-analysis. *Journal of Family Psychology*, 15, 355–370.

Amato, P.R. (2014). The consequences of divorce for adults and children: An update. *Drustvena istrazivanja: Journal for General Social Issues*, 23(1), 5–24. https://doi.org/10.5559/di.5523.5551.5501.

Amato, P.R. & Cheadle, J. (2005). The long reach of divorce: Divorce and child well-being across three generations. *Journal of Marriage and Family*, 67(1), 191–206.

Amato, P.R. & Keith, B. (1991). Parental divorce and the well-being of children: A meta-analysis. *Psychological Bulletin*, 110(1), 25–46.

Anderson, S.R., Anderson, S.A., Palmer, K.L., Mutchler, M.S. & Baker, L.K. (2010). Defining high conflict. *The American Journal of Family Therapy*, 39, 11–27. https://doi.org/10.1080/01926187.2010.530194.

Andrews, B., Brewin, C.R., Philpott, R. & Stewart, L. (2007). Delayed-onset posttraumatic stress disorder: A systematic review of the evidence. *American Journal of Psychiatry*, 164(9), 1319–1326.

Asen, E. & Morris, E. (2016). Making contact happen in chronic litigation cases: A mentalizing approach. *Family Law*, April 2016: 511–515.

Bateson, G. (1972). *Steps to an Ecology of Mind: Collected Essays in Anthropology, Psychiatry, Evolution, and Epistemology*. Chicago: University of Chicago Press.

Baumeister, R.F., Bratslavsky, E., Finkenauer, C. & Vohs, K.D. (2001). Bad is stronger than good. *Review of General Psychology*, 5(4), 323–370.

Berne, E. (1964). *Games People Play*. New York: Grove Press.

Bernet, W., Boch-Galgau, W. von, Baker, A.J.L. & Morrison, S.L. (2010). Parental alienation, DSM-V, and ICD-11. *The American Journal of Family Therapy*, 38, 176–187.

Boss, P. (2006). *Loss, Trauma and Resilience. Therapeutic Work with Ambiguous Loss*. New York: Norton.

Bradbury, T.N. & Fincham, F.D. (1992). Attributions and behavior in Marital Interaction. *Journal of Personality and Social Psychology*, 63, 613–628.

Bream, V. & Buchanan, A. (2003). Distress among children whose separated or divorced parents cannot agree arrangements for them. *British Journal of Social Work*, 33, 227–238.

Buehler, C. & Gerard, J.M. (2002). Marital conflict, ineffective parenting, and children's and adolescents' maladjustment. *Journal of Marriage and Family*, 64, 78–92.

Bushman, B.J. & Baumeister, R.F. (1998). Threatened egotism, narcissism, self-esteem, and direct and displaced aggression: Does self-love or self-hate lead to violence? *Journal of Personality and Social Psychology*, 75, 219–229.

Buysse, A., Put, J., Rober, P., Schoors, K., Taelman, P. & Verschelden, G. (2011). *Is er een goede manier om te scheiden? Interdisciplinair onderzoek naar optimalisatie van scheidingstrajecten*. Universiteit van Gent/Katholieke Universiteit Leuven: IPOS.

Byng-Hall, J. (1985). The family script: A useful bridge between theory and practice. *Journal of Family Therapy*, 7, 301–305.

Cashmore, J.A. & Parkinson, P.N. (2011). Reasons for disputes in high conflict families. *Journal of Family Studies*, 17, 186–203.

Chen, E. & Miller, G.E. (2012). "Shift-and-persist" strategies why low socioeconomic status isn't always bad for health. *Perspectives on Psychological Science*, 7(2), 135–158.

Cohen, J.A., Mannarino, A.P., Kliethermes, M. & Murray, L.A. (2012). Trauma-focused CBT for youth with complex trauma. *Child Abuse & Neglect*, 36(6), 528–541.

Cohen, J.A., Mannarino, A.P. & Murray, L.K. (2011). Trauma-focused CBT for youth who experience ongoing traumas. *Child Abuse & Neglect*, 35(8), 637–646.

Cohen, S. & Wills, T.A. (1985). Stress, social support, and the buffering hypothesis. *Psychological Bulletin*, 98, 310–357.

Cottyn, L. (2009). Conflicten tussen ouders na scheiding. *Systeemtheoretisch Bulletin*, XXVII, 2.

Dalton, C., Carbon, S. & Olesen, N. (2003). High conflict divorce, violence, and abuse: Implications for custody and visitation decisions. *Juvenile and Family Court Journal*, 54, 11–33.

Davies, P.T., Winter, M.A. & Cicchetti, D. (2006). The implications of emotional security theory for understanding and treating childhood psychopathology. *Development and Psychopathology*, 18, 707–735.

Decety, J. & Jackson, P.L. (2004). The functional architecture of human empathy. *Behavioral and Cognitive Neuroscience Reviews*, 3, 71–100.

De Los Reyes, A. & Kazdin, A.E. (2005). Informant discrepancies in the assessment of childhood psychopathology: A critical review, theoretical framework, and recommendations for further study. *Psychological Bulletin*, 131(4), 483–509.

Diehl, M. & Hay, E.L. (2010). Risk and resilience factors in coping with daily stress in adulthood: The role of age, self-concept incoherence, and personal control. *Developmental Psychology*, 46(5), 1132–1146.

Dijkstra, S. & Verhoeven, W. (2014). Ouderschap na scheiding en geweld met dodelijke afloop. *Gescheiden werelden en gespannen verhoudingen.* Maatwerk vakblad voor maatschappelijk werk, 2–6.

Dullaert, M. (2014). *Vechtende ouders, het kind in de knel – Adviesrapport over het verbeteren van de positie van kinderen in vechtscheidingen.* Den Haag: Bureau Nationale ombudsman. Te vinden op www.dekinderombudsman.nl/ul/cms/fck-uploaded/KOM003.2014Kinderombudsmanadviesrapportvechtscheidingen.pdf

Exline, J.J., Baumeister, R.F., Bushman, B.J., Campbell, W.K. & Finkel, E.J. (2004). Too proud to let go: Narcissistic entitlement as a barrier to forgiveness. *Journal of Personality and Social Psychology*, 87, 894–912.

Fincham, F.D. & Beach, S.R.H. (1999). Conflict in marriage: Implications for working with couples. *Annual Review of Psychology*, 50, 47–77.

Fincham, F.D. & Bradbury, T.N. (1987). Cognitive processes and conflict in close relationships: An attribution-efficacy model. *Journal of Personality and Social Psychology*, 53(6), 1106.

Finkenauer, C., Kluwer, E.S., Kroese, J.H. & Visser, M. (2018). Trust as an antidote to the co-parenting conflict in high-conflict divorce relationships. In: Bertoni, A., Donato, S. & Molgora, S. (eds.), *When "We" Are Stressed: A Dyadic Approach to Coping with Stressful Events*, pp. 87–105. Hauppauge, NY: Nova Science Publishers. ISBN: 9781536133509.

Finkenauer, C., Visser, M., Schoemaker, K. & de Kruijff, A. (2017). Kenmerken van vechtscheidende gezinnen: Een beschrijvend onderzoek naar ouders en kinderen die verwikkeld zijn in een vechtscheiding. *Tijdschrift voor Orthopedagogiek*, 56, 444–458.

Fonagy, P., Gergeley, G., Jurist, E. et al. (2002). *Affect Regulation, Mentalisation and the Development of the Self.* New York: Other Press.

Fotheringham, S., Dunbar, J. & Hensley, D. (2013). Speaking for themselves: Hope for children caught in high conflict custody and access disputes involving domestic violence. *Journal of Family Violence*, 28, 311–324.

Frederickson, B. (2009). *Positivity: Discover the Upward Spiral that Will Change Your Life*.

Friedman, R.A. & Currall, S.C. (2003). Conflict escalation: Dispute exacerbating elements of e-mail communication. *Human Relations*, 56(11), 1325–1347.

Friese, M., Hofmann, W. & Wiers, R.W. (2011). On taming horses and strengthening riders: Recent developments in research on interventions to improve self-control in health behaviors. *Self and Identity*, 10(3), 336–351.

Gardner, R.A. (1998). *The Parental Alienation Syndrome: A Guide for Mental Health and Legal Professionals* (2nd ed.). Creskill, NJ: CreativeTherapeutics.

Gere, J. & Schimmack, U. (2013). When romantic partners' goals conflict: Effects on relationship quality and subjective well-being. *Journal of Happiness Studies*, 14, 37–49.

Glasl, F. (2001). *Help! Conflicten: heb ik een conflict, of heeft het conflict mij?* Zeist: Christofoor.

Gollwitzer, P.M. & Brandstatter, V. (1997). Implementation intentions and effective goal pursuit. *Journal of Personality and Social Psychology*, 73, 186–199.

Gottman, J.M. (1998). Psychology and the study of marital processes. *Annual Review of Psychology*, 49(1), 169–197.

Greenstein, T.N. (2009). National context, family satisfaction, and fairness in the division of household labor. *Journal of Marriage and Family*, 71, 1039–1051.

Groen, M. (2013). Spanningen tussen twee systemen: zorg en recht. In: Groen, M. & van Lawick, M.J. (Red.), *Intieme oorlog. Over de kwetsbaarheid van familierelaties*. Amsterdam: Van Gennep.

Guven, C., Senik, C. & Stichnoth, H. (2012). You can't be happier than your wife. Happiness gaps and divorce. *Journal of Economic Behavior & Organization*, 82, 110–130.

Harnett, P.H. (2007). A procedure for assessing parents' capacity for change in child protection cases. *Children and Youth Services Review*, 29, 1179–1188.

Hennik, R. van & Hillewaere, B. (2017). Practice based evidence based practice – Navigating based on coordinated improvisation, collaborative learning and multimethods research in Feedback Informed Systemic Therapy. *Journal of Family Therapy*, 39(3), 288–309.

Hetherington, E.M. & Elmore, A.M. (2003). Risk and resilience in children coping with their parents' divorce and remarriage. *Resilience and Vulnerability: Adaptation in the Context of Childhood Adversities*, 182–212.

Hughes, K. (2005). The adult children of divorce – Pure relationships and family values? *Journal of Sociology*, 42, 69–86.

Hurst, M. (2011). Professional judgement in the assessment of risk: Is there a role for systemic practice? *Journal of Family Therapy*, 33, 168–180.

Jaffe, P.G., Crooks, C.V. & Poisson, S.E. (2003). Common misconceptions in addressing domestic violence in child custody disputes. *Juvenile and Family Court Journal*, 54, 57–67.

Johnston, J.R. (1994). High conflict divorce. *Children and Divorce*, 4, 165–182.

Johnston, J.R. (2006). The psychological functioning of alienated children and their parents in custody disputing families: A program of research. Paper presented at *the International Conference on Children and Divorce*, 24–27 July 2006. University of East Anglia, Norwich, UK.

Jonge, A.L.J. de, Van, H.L. & Peen, J. (2013). De rol van patiëntkenmerken bij indicatiestelling voor psychodynamische psychotherapie. *Tijdschrift voor psychiatrie*, 55(1), 35–44.

Kelly, J.B. & Emery, R.E. (2003). Children's adjustment following divorce: Risk and resilience perspectives. *Family Relations*, 52(4), 352–362. https://doi.org/10.1111/j.1741-3729.2003.00352.x

Kelly, J.B. & Johnston, J.R. (2001). The alienated child: A reformulation of parental alienation syndrome. *Family and Conciliation Courts Review*, 39, 249–266.

Kluwer, E.S., Heesink, J.A.M. & Vliert, E. van de (2002). The division of labor across the transition to parenthood: A justice perspective. *Journal of Marriage and Family*, 64, 930–943.

Lagattuta, K.H., Sayfan, L. & Bamford, C. (2012). Do you know how I feel? Parents underestimate worry and overestimate optimism compared to child self-report. *Journal of Experimental Child Psychology*, 113(2), 211–232.

Lang, P.J. (1985). The cognitive psychophysiology of emotion: Fear and anxiety. In: Tuma, A.H. & Maser, J.D. (Eds.), *Anxiety and the Anxiety Disorders*. Hillsdale: Lawrence Erlbaum.

Lawick, J. van (2012). Vechtscheidende ouders en hun kinderen. *Systeemtherapie*, 24, 129–150.

Lazarus, R.S. & Folkman, S. (1984). *Stress, Appraisal, and Coping*. New York: Springer.

Lebow, J. & Rekart, K.N. (2007). Integrative family therapy for high-conflict divorce with disputes over child custody and visitation. *Family Process*, 46, 79–91.

López-Pérez, B. & Wilson, E.L. (2015). Parent-child discrepancies in the assessment of children's and adolescents' happiness. *Journal of Experimental Child Psychology*, 139, 249–255.

Maccoby, E. & Mnookin, R.H. (1992). *Dividing the Child: Social and Legal Dilemmas of Custody*. Cambridge, MA: Harvard University Press.

Mason, B. (1993). Towards positions of safe uncertainty. *The Journal of Systemic Consultation & Management*, 4, 189–200.

Masten, A.S. & Narayan, A.J. (2012). Child development in the context of disaster, war, and terrorism: Pathways of risk and resilience. *Psychology*, 63.

Meulen, L. Van der (2017). *Kinderen uit de Knel; ervaringen van Vlaamse Hulpverleners. Masterthese*. KU Leuven: Instituut voor familiale en seksuologische wetenschappen.

Middelberg, C.V. (2001). Projective identification in common couple dances. *Journal of Marital and Family Therapy*, 27, 341–352.

Olthof, J. (2012). *Handboek Narratieve Psychotherapie*. Utrecht: De Tijdstroom.

Omer, H. (2007). *Geweldloos verzet in gezinnen. Een nieuwe benadering van gewelddadig en zelfdestructief gedrag van kinderen en adolescenten*. Houten: Bohn Stafleu van Loghum.

Oppenheim, D. (2006). Child, parent, and parent–child emotion narratives: Implications for developmental psychopathology. *Development and Psychopathology*, 18(3), 771–790.

Parys, H. van, Bonnewyn, A., Hooghe, A., De Mol, J. & Rober, P. (2015). Toward understanding the child's experience in the process of parentification: Young adults' reflections on growing up with a depressed parent. *Journal of Marital and Family Therapy*, 41(4), 522–536.

Pels, T., Lünnemann, K. & Steketee, M. (Red.). (2011). *Opvoeden na partnergeweld. Ondersteuning van moeders en jongeren van diverse afkomst*. Assen: Van Gorcum.

Pinedo, M. & Vollinga, P. (2013). *Aan alle gescheiden ouders. Leer kijken door de ogen van je kind*. Utrecht: Bruna Uitgevers.

Rhmaty, F. (2011). *Transculturele traumaverwerking met vluchtelingen*. Assen: van Gorcum.

Ridley, C.A., Wilhelm, M.S., & Surra, C.A. (2001). Married couples' conflict responses and marital quality. *Journal of Social and Personal Relationships*, 18, 517–534.

Rober, P. (2012). *De praktijk van de gezinstherapie*. Leuven: Acco.

Rusbult, C.E. & Van Lange, P.A.M. (2003). Interdependence, interaction, and relationships. *Annual Review of Psychology*, 54, 351–375.

Savenije, A., Lawick, M.J. van & Reijmers, E.T.M. (2014). *Handboek Systeemtherapie*. Utrecht: De Tijdstroom.

Scheinkman, M. & Dekoven Fishbane, M. (2004). The vulnerability cycle – Working with impasses in couple therapy. *Family Process*, 45(3), 279–299.

Schoemaker, K., Kruijff, A. de, Visser, M., Lawick, J. van & Finkenauer, C. (2017). *Vechtscheidingen. Beleving en ervaringen van ouders en Kinderen en verandering na Kinderen uit de Knel*. Onderzoeksrapport. Academische Werkplaats aanpak Kindermishandeling.

Schoen, R. & Canudas-Romo, V. (2006). Timing effects on divorce: 20th century experience in the United States. *Journal of Marriage and Family*, 68(3), 749–758.

Showers, C.J. & Zeigler-Hill, V. (2007). Compartmentalization and integration: The evaluative organization of contextualized selves. *Journal of Personality*, 75(6), 1181–1204.

Siegel, M.D. (2012). *The Developing Mind: How Relationships and the Brain Interact to Shape Who We Are*. New York: Guilford.

Spillane-Grieco, E. (2000). Cognitive-behavioral family therapy with a family in high-conflict divorce: A case study. *Clinical Social Work Journal*, 28, 105–119.

Spruijt, E. & Kormos, H. (2014). *Handboek Scheiden en de kinderen. Voor de beroepskracht die met scheidingskinderen te maken heeft. Tweede herziene druk*. Houten: Bohn Stafleu van Loghum.

Steuber, K.R. & Solomon, D.H. (2011). Factors that predict married partners' disclosures about infertility to social network members. *Journal of Applied Communication Research*, 39, 250–270.

Treutler, C.M. & Epkins, C.C. (2003). Are discrepancies among child, mother, and father reports on children's behavior related to parents' psychological symptoms and aspects of parent–child relationships? *Journal of Abnormal Child Psychology*, 31(1), 13–27.

van der Elst, E., Wierstra, J., Lawick, J. Van & Visser, M. (in press). *Group Therapy for High-Conflict Divorce: A Workbook for the "No Kids in the Middle" Intervention Program.* Abingdon: Routledge.

Vangelisti, A., Knapp, M.L. & Daly, J.A. (1990). Conversational narcissism. *Communication Monographs*, 251–274.

Verheugt, A.J. (2007). *Moordouders. Kinderdoding in Nederland: een klinisch en forensisch psychologische studie naar de persoon van de kinderdoder.* Assen: Van Gorcum.

Visser, M., Finkenauer, C., Schoemaker, K., Kluwer, E., Rijken, van der, R., Lawick, van J., Bom, H., Schipper, de J.C. & Lamers-Winkelman, F. (2017). I'll never forgive you: High conflict divorce, social network, and co-parenting conflicts. *Journal of Child and Family Studies*, 26(11), 3055–3066.

Voert, M.ter. (2019). *Scheidingen 2018. Gerechtelijke procedures en gesubsidieerde rechtsbijstand.* Geraadpleegd van www.wodc.nl/binaries.

Vreeswijk, van, M.F., Broersen, J., & Nadort, M. (2008). *Handboek schematherapie*. Houten: Bohn Stafleu van Loghum.

Wal, R.C. Van der, Finkenauer, C. & Visser, M.M. (2019). Reconciling mixed findings on children's adjustment following high-conflict divorce. *Journal of Child and Family Studies*, 28(2), 468–478.

Wallerstein, J.S. (1986). Women after divorce – Preliminary-report from a 10-year follow-up. *American Journal of Orthopsychiatry*, 56, 65–77.

Whiteside, M.F. (1998). The parental alliance following divorce: An overview. *Journal of Marital and Family Therapy*, 24(1), 3–24. https://doi.org/10.1111/j.1752-0606.1998.tb01060.x

Whiteside, M.F. & Becker, B.J. (2000). Parental factors and the young child's postdivorce adjustment: A meta-analysis with implications for parenting arrangements. *Journal of Family Psychology*, 14(1), 5. https://doi.org/10.1037/0893-3200.14.1.5.

Wildschut, T., Pinter, B., Vevea, J.L., Insko, C.A. & Schopler, J. (2003). Beyond the group mind: A quantitative review of the interindividual-intergroup discontinuity effect. *Psychological Bulletin*, 129, 698–722.

Wilson, J. (2007). *The Performance of Practice: Enhancing the Repertoire of Therapy with Children and Families*. London: Karnac.

Zander, J. (2011). Ouderverstoting en de vergeten vaderlijke opvoedingsverantwoordelijkheid. *Pedagogiek*, 31, 103–113.

For Product Safety Concerns and Information please contact our EU
representative GPSR@taylorandfrancis.com
Taylor & Francis Verlag GmbH, Kaufingerstraße 24, 80331 München, Germany

www.ingramcontent.com/pod-product-compliance
Ingram Content Group UK Ltd.
Pitfield, Milton Keynes, MK11 3LW, UK
UKHW020130200926
475702UK00005B/684
9780367109226